Awaken with Methylene Blue

The Ultimate Guide to
Ignite Cognitive & Physical Performance,
Optimize Mitochondria & Cellular Health,
And Extend Your Healthspan

Nova L. Phoenix

Contents

Introduction

New Kind of Blue

There's a reason methylene blue is captivating the curiosity of both scientists and longevity seekers alike. In these times, we aspire for sharper minds, stronger bodies, and deeper reserves of vitality. This powerful blue molecule is quietly emerging as a potent ally and is making waves in the wellness community.

Initially discovered in the 19th century as a dye, methylene blue's journey from textile to therapeutic is as unexpected as it is inspiring. What began as a laboratory stain has evolved into something far more impactful: a compound that holds promise for protecting brain cells, enhancing mitochondrial function, improving mental clarity, and potentially extending the human healthspan. This guide was created not just to share facts but to empower your exploration. What follows isn't about one person's authority; it's about weaving together credible science, clinical history, and lived experiences so you can discover what resonates for you.

Whether you're a biohacker seeking to supercharge your brain and cellular edge, a longevity enthusiast aiming to repair mitochondrial damage and slow aging from the inside out, a practitioner supporting clients with neurodegenerative concerns, a fitness seeker wanting faster recovery and deeper performance gains, or simply someone looking to feel more alive in your own body, this book is for you.

Inside, you'll find practical protocols, guidance on integrating it into your daily life, safety guidelines, and real-life stories of transformation. But more than that, you'll find a framework for working with methylene blue as a conscious tool that invites you to listen to your body, honor your intuition, and work in harmony with your cells rather than against them. We'll begin by anchoring in the foundational science, exploring how methylene blue works within the mitochondria and nervous system to support energy, clarity, and resilience. From there, we'll delve into protocols, supplement stacks, personalized usage tips, debunking myths, and even speculative frontiers that hint at where this molecule may be headed next.

But this is not just about optimization for the sake of productivity. This is about coming home to yourself; clearer, calmer, more present. This is about remembering that healing and performance are not separate; they are two expressions of a body in balance.

Energy is life's currency, and every moment you wait is a moment your cells keep operating below their potential. The shift can begin as soon as you allow it. Welcome to *The Blue*

Biohack. You're not just here to learn. You're here to awaken. So, let's begin with the unexpected journey of this blue molecule.

Chapter 1

The Origins and Awakening of Methylene Blue

Few compounds have traveled such a winding and wondrous road in the journey through medical history as methylene blue. Born in the late 1800s as a fabric dye, this bold blue molecule soon found its way into microscopes, medicine bottles, and eventually into the hands of biohackers, scientists, and seekers of vitality. What began as a tool to color cloth evolved into a tool to illuminate human potential, both literally and energetically.

A Color That Changed Medicine

Methylene blue first made scientific waves for its ability to stain living cells, granting researchers new visibility into the microscopic world. For the first time, cellular structures were no longer hidden in the shadows; they were vivid, defined, and full of insight. This advancement helped unlock discoveries in biology, pathology, and hematology, catalyzing a deeper understanding of the body's inner workings.

Not long after, methylene blue proved it could do more than reveal. It could heal.

Neuroscientist Francisco Gonzalez-Lima has been a leading voice in showing how methylene blue can enhance memory and brain energy metabolism. His findings, echoed by other researchers and by lived experience in the wellness community, are part of what makes this molecule's revival so compelling.

Even long before modern neuroscience, methylene blue was proving its value in medicine. In the early 20th century, Nobel Prize-winning physician Paul Ehrlich famously used it as one of the first synthetic drugs to treat malaria. It offered a synthetic solution to combat a historically lethal disease. This marked a pivotal shift, proving that methylene blue was more than just a colorful lab compound and demonstrating its versatile adaptation to human needs. It was a bridge between early pharmacology and the modern era of targeted medicine.

During World War II, due to its antimicrobial properties, methylene blue was employed to treat urinary tract infections. Later, its impact broadened beyond infectious disease into the realm of psychiatric treatment with the development of phenothiazine antipsychotics, early psychiatric medications that shaped the course of mental health treatment in the 20th century.

Today, methylene blue is FDA-approved for treating methemoglobinemia, a condition that limits the blood's ability to carry oxygen. It is also still used as a trusted surgical dye. Its adaptability, strong safety record, and unique ability to influence multiple cellular processes continue to capture the attention of researchers worldwide.

This molecule's story is one of transformation and repurposing, an invitation to consider how something old can become revolutionary when seen with new eyes.

A Modern Resurgence

Today, methylene blue is experiencing a revival. Biohackers celebrate its ability to enhance energy, mood, and focus. Holistic practitioners recognize its impact on mitochondrial health and oxidative stress. Longevity seekers see its potential to slow aging at the cellular level. Athletes turn to it for faster recovery and enhanced endurance.

Why? At its core, methylene blue helps the body function as it was designed to, producing energy more efficiently. And in a world where many are exhausted, inflamed, or burned out, that energy is everything.

Its appeal is universal. Whether you're a high-performing entrepreneur, a curious healer, or someone simply looking to feel better in your body and brain, methylene blue offers a bridge between ancient wisdom and modern optimization.

Unveiling Broader Possibilities

As methylene blue transitioned from the lab to therapeutic use, its reach expanded far beyond what scientists initially envisioned. It helped shape the early understanding of neurotransmitters and brain chemistry, ultimately contributing to the development of medications that transformed psychiatric care.

Today, its potential continues to surprise. In addition to its use in treating conditions like carbon monoxide and cyanide poisoning, it's being explored for its role in improving memory, preventing neurodegeneration, and even as a complementary tool in cancer therapy.

Methylene blue is one of the most intriguing compounds in integrative health today because of its adaptability. It crosses boundaries between diagnostics, detoxification, and cognitive enhancement.

This chapter isn't just a walk through history; it's a glimpse into the soul of a substance that continues to evolve in tandem with human consciousness.

Reflective Invitation: Where Are You on the Map?

Pause for a moment and reflect.

- When did your health journey begin?
- What drew you to explore outside the mainstream?
- Where do you feel depleted? Where do you long to feel more alive?

Let methylene blue be a conversation starter between your body and your potential; a tool, not a fix, that you can use to explore your inner vitality.

Journal Prompt:

- What qualities do I hope to awaken through this journey, mentally, physically, and emotionally?
- What would it look like to feel truly energized?

Mitochondria and the Mechanics of Energy

To understand why methylene blue is so powerful, we need to zoom in on the mitochondria, the cellular engines that produce ATP, the fuel for nearly everything your body does.

Methylene blue helps these engines run cleaner and more efficiently. It can bypass broken steps in the electron transport chain, restore balance to redox reactions, and reduce the oxidative stress that leads to aging and fatigue.

In short, it doesn't just support energy; it helps rewire how your body creates and protects it.

Methylene blue's neuroprotective properties have ignited considerable interest, mainly due to its effects on brain health. Beyond preserving neuron energy efficiency, it prevents the accumulation of misfolded proteins, a common feature in neurodegenerative diseases such as Alzheimer's. By stabilizing these protein formations, methylene blue may potentially halt the progression of devastating disorders, offering hope for neuroprotection. This cornerstone attribute contributes to maintaining cognitive functions by ensuring neurons have the necessary energy for complex mental operations.

And because mitochondrial health is linked to brain function, inflammation, immune balance, and longevity, supporting this system creates a ripple effect that touches every cell.

Hypothetical Example: Cognitive Upgrade in Action

Imagine a creative professional, let's call her Jessica, who struggles with mental fatigue and late-afternoon brain fog. She begins incorporating a microdose of methylene blue into her routine, starting low and slow, as outlined in later chapters.

Over time, Jessica notices more sustained focus during deep work sessions. Her ideas come more easily. She's less reactive under pressure and more resilient to daily stress. She pairs her use of methylene blue with light movement and breathwork, amplifying her results. Is methylene blue the only factor in Jessica's upgrade? No. But it acts as a catalyst, allowing her body's own systems to function with more clarity, energy, and ease.

A Blueprint for What's Possible

Methylene blue's potential extends beyond the individual. It also represents a merging of traditional medicine and contemporary biohacking. Whether boosting cognitive performance or enhancing cellular vitality, methylene blue offers a scientifically backed approach to achieving remarkable health outcomes across various life situations. This duality reflects the blend of past knowledge with present innovations, promising continued breakthroughs for those willing to delve further into its multifaceted benefits.

Methylene blue is not a magic pill but a deeply intelligent molecule. Its ability to adapt across therapeutic domains, support mitochondrial function, and protect the brain makes it one of the most promising biohacking tools of our time.

As you read this book, let your curiosity be your guide. The science will deepen, and the applications will become more personalized.

But for now, know this: methylene blue has been waiting. And you've just begun to unlock what it can offer.

In the chapters ahead, we'll move step by step, beginning with the foundational science of how methylene blue works, then into safe and effective usage, daily integration practices, and the more advanced possibilities that are emerging. For now, take a simple baseline: write down one word that describes how your body feels today, and one word that captures how you long to feel. Hold onto these words. They will serve as a compass as we continue this journey together.

Chapter 2

The Health Benefits of Methylene Blue

Fueling Focus, Vitality, and Longevity from the Inside Out

Most of us want to feel more alive, clearer in thought, stronger in body, and more energized throughout the day. Methylene blue offers a path to that vitality by working at the most fundamental level of our biology: the mitochondria.

These tiny power plants inside our cells are responsible for producing the energy that fuels everything from our brainpower to our physical stamina. And methylene blue? It acts like an energetic amplifier, optimizing how mitochondria perform and protecting them from the wear and tear of stress, aging, and disease.

This chapter examines the key benefits of methylene blue, including its support for cognitive function, protection against aging, reduction of oxidative stress, enhancement of oxygen utilization, and restoration of mitochondrial health.

Enhancing Cognitive Function: Focus, Clarity, and Brain Resilience

Imagine starting your morning with a clear, focused mind, calm yet sharp, alert without tension. That's one of the first changes many users report after incorporating methylene blue into their routine.

Methylene blue enhances ATP production in brain cells by improving mitochondrial efficiency, leading to improved mental stamina, sharper focus, and enhanced memory. It also crosses the blood-brain barrier, allowing it to act directly on neuronal tissues to support clarity and learning.

Scientific research supports these claims. One placebo-controlled study showed that a single low dose of methylene blue significantly improved memory retention and visual recall in healthy adults during cognitive tasks. Another study suggests it may enhance connectivity between brain regions involved in memory processing, making it a powerful nootropic ally.

This can result in reduced mental fatigue, better decision-making, and the ability to stay "in the zone" longer. Lisa, a medical student who began microdosing methylene blue before exam season, described it this way: *"It was like my brain stopped glitching. I could study longer, but I could also study better. It felt like everything just clicked."*

Reflective Prompt:

When do you feel most mentally drained or scattered?

How would increased focus change the quality of your work or your life?

Anti-Aging: Cellular Longevity and Radiance

The aging process isn't just about wrinkles or slowing down. At its core, aging is about the accumulation of damage at the cellular level, and particularly damage to the mitochondria. When these engines falter, the entire system begins to slow. Methylene blue helps counteract that. Improving mitochondrial function and reducing oxidative stress helps preserve cellular integrity and delay biological aging. It even stimulates collagen and elastin production in the skin, improving texture and elasticity.

In a study published in *Scientific Reports*, human skin cells treated with methylene blue exhibited increased hydration, reduced signs of aging, and enhanced antioxidant activity. Beyond the skin, researchers have found evidence that methylene blue can extend lifespan in animal models by supporting mitochondrial resilience and decreasing DNA damage.

For those committed to graceful aging, it's a tool that works from the inside out. Sarah, a holistic health coach in her sixties, shares: *"It's not about looking young, it's about feeling vibrant. Methylene blue has become part of how I care for my energy, my mind, and my skin."*

Try This:

Add a few drops of methylene blue to your morning routine (under guidance), then journal how your energy, focus, and skin feel after one week, one month, and one season.

Oxidative Stress: Calming the Cellular Storm

Our modern lives expose us to toxins, stress, processed food, and EMFs. All of which increase oxidative stress in the body. This internal imbalance leads to inflammation, fatigue, chronic illness, accelerated aging, and cellular damage. Methylene blue is unique among antioxidants. It doesn't just scavenge free radicals; it prevents their formation by optimizing how mitochondria breathe. By donating electrons in the electron transport chain, it reduces the chance of electron "leakage" and the creation of reactive oxygen species (ROS). This makes it both a firefighter and a fire preventer.

Its protective qualities are essential for the brain, which is highly sensitive to oxidative damage. But they also support the heart, muscles, skin, and immune system: athletes using methylene blue report faster recovery, reduced soreness, and improved endurance.

It's like giving your cells a shield and a boost at the same time: protection + energy. But oxidative stress doesn't only come from physical exertion; it's also the result of emotional stress, toxic exposures, and poor sleep. Methylene blue acts as a calming influence on the cellular level, bringing order to inner chaos.

Mitochondrial Repair: The Blueprint for Vital Energy

Healthy mitochondria = healthy cells. And methylene blue's unique mechanism of donating and shuttling electrons helps restore optimal mitochondrial function, especially when damage has already occurred.

One study in animal models found that methylene blue improved mitochondrial respiration and stabilized mitochondrial membrane potential, which are key indicators of cellular energy production. This kind of repair is foundational for sustained vitality, especially as we age or face chronic stress.

Whether you're navigating long hours at work, recovering from illness, or simply seeking to feel more "switched on," supporting your mitochondria is one of the most efficient ways to elevate your health. Methylene blue is one of the few compounds that can do that both preventatively and therapeutically.

Reflection Prompt

How often do you feel fully energized?

What if your vitality was no longer fragile, but steady and sustained?

Oxygen Optimization: Breathing New Life Into Every Cell

Each breath you take offers life to your cells, but how well do they receive it? Methylene blue enhances oxygen utilization, helping your mitochondria make the most of every inhale. This becomes especially valuable during physical exertion, altitude changes, or fatigue.

Studies have explored its application in improving aerobic capacity and protecting against altitude sickness. However, even outside of extremes, its benefits can be felt in day-to-day life, including increased stamina during workouts, quicker recovery, and sharper mental performance.

By improving mitochondrial efficiency, methylene blue also reduces metabolic waste, leaving your cells with more energy and fewer byproducts. It's not just about adding oxygen, but it's also about using what you already have better.

Reflective Prompt

Are you breathing through your life or rushing through it?

How might optimized oxygenation shift your capacity, presence, and ease?

Final Thoughts: Returning to Vitality

Methylene blue is not a magic pill. It's a molecular ally, a partner in reclaiming energy, protecting longevity, and living life from a more bottomless well of vitality.

By supporting mitochondrial health, enhancing oxygen utilization, and shielding against oxidative stress, methylene blue helps us regain our radiance. And not as an escape from aging or exhaustion, but as a reminder that our body *wants* to heal. It wants to thrive.

This molecule simply reminds us how.

Summary Snapshot: Why Methylene Blue?

Let's recap. Methylene blue offers:

- Enhanced focus, memory, and mental clarity
- Protection against aging at the cellular level
- Powerful antioxidant support against oxidative stress
- Mitochondrial repair and energy production
- Improved oxygen use and physical performance

It accomplishes all of this while working in harmony with the body, not against it. This isn't about quick fixes. It's about tuning into your energy, protecting your longevity, and upgrading your health from the inside out.

Chapter 3

Safe and Effective Usage Guidelines

Imagine yourself as a skilled navigator, charting a course through the vast sea of supplements, and methylene blue is the beacon of promise on the horizon. This chapter will equip you with the essential knowledge to use methylene blue safely, effectively, and harmoniously, taking into account your unique biology.

Personalized dosing is key. Your physiology, including your age, weight, health status, and personal goals, all influence how you respond to methylene blue. A one-size-fits-all approach does not apply in this case. Even among people with similar intentions, differences in lifestyle, genetics, and internal chemistry can lead to very different outcomes. That is why personalization is not just ideal, it is necessary. It helps you unlock the full benefits of methylene blue while minimizing potential risks.

Methylene blue is available in several forms. Oral tablets and capsules are convenient and easy to incorporate into daily routines. Sublingual (held under the tongue) allows faster absorption into the bloodstream and a quicker onset of effects. This option is advantageous when seeking an immediate cognitive lift or energy surge. Liquid drops, on the other hand, offer unmatched flexibility, allowing for fine-tuned adjustments in dosage. Some days call for the long-lasting steadiness of a capsule, while other days may benefit from the immediacy of a sublingual or liquid dose. Each method is a tool in your wellness toolkit, and how and when you use them depends on your needs and your rhythm.

To determine your ideal dose, begin by clarifying your health goals, whether it is a cognitive enhancement, a boost in energy, or cellular support for healthy aging. Then, consider your body weight, which plays a significant role in how your body processes supplements. A general starting range is 0.5–1 mg per kilogram of body weight (or approximately 0.23–0.45 mg per pound). For example, someone weighing 150 pounds (68 kg) might start with a dose between 34 - 68 mg. Always begin at the lower end of the range and gradually increase as needed, ideally with the guidance of a knowledgeable practitioner. The adage "start low and go slow" is not just wise but strategic. Starting with a low dose and gradually increasing it allows your body to adapt, giving you space to observe how methylene blue affects you. Your response can vary depending on factors such as sleep, diet, and stress. Hence, listening to your body along the way is essential. Moving slowly and intentionally reduces the risk of side effects while discovering the sweet spot where benefits are maximized and your system remains balanced.

Interactive Exercise: Crafting Your Dosage Plan

To bring the theoretical knowledge into practice, let us engage in an interactive exercise designed to help you create a personalized dosage plan.

Define Your Goals: Identify the benefits you aim to achieve with methylene blue and write down your primary objectives.

Assess Your Baseline: Consider your current energy levels and mental acuity. Jot down any pre-existing conditions or medications that might influence methylene blue's efficacy, including allergies or sensitivities. This step is crucial as it helps identify potential interactions or contraindications, and will be discussed in more detail in the chapters to come.

Choose Your Delivery Method: Based on your convenience and preference, select the delivery method that suits you best: tablets, sublingual drops, or liquid forms. Your lifestyle might influence this choice. For example, busy mornings could lean towards tablets, while more flexible days might see you experimenting with liquid drops or the immediacy of sublingual options.

Calculate the Initial Dose: Use the guideline of 0.23-0.45 mg/lb. (0.5-1 mg per kilogram.) of body weight. Adjust according to your goals and any professional guidance you receive. Maintain flexibility; while the initial plan is a foundation, adaptability is key as you progress and respond.

Monitor and Adjust: Document your experiences and any symptomatic changes or side effects. Adjust your dose as necessary based on your experiences.

Maintain a journal to track the physical and cognitive effects, refining your plan continuously. This record will prove invaluable in recognizing patterns and making informed adjustments.

You cultivate a tailored plan aligned with your unique needs and health goals by following these steps. This process is dynamic; feel free to adjust it based on your experiences and feedback from healthcare professionals. A personalized dosage plan helps you achieve optimal results while prioritizing safety and efficacy.

Table 1: Dosage ~ Guide by Weight & Intent

Weight (lbs)	Longevity / Anti-Aging (0.25–0.5 mg/ kg)	Cognitive Enhancement (0.5–1 mg/kg)	Athletic Performance* (0.5–1 mg/kg)
100	11–23 mg	23–45 mg	23–45 mg
120	14–27 mg	27–55 mg	27–55 mg
140	16–32 mg	32–64 mg	32–64 mg
160	18–36 mg	36–73 mg	36–73 mg
180	20–41 mg	41–82 mg	41–82 mg
200	23–45 mg	45–91 mg	45–91 mg
220	25–50 mg	50–100 mg	50–100 mg
240	27–55 mg	55–109 mg	55–109 mg

While these ranges offer useful guidance, many people benefit from starting even lower and gradually adjusting upward as needed.

*Athletic Performance is listed at the same range as Cognitive Enhancement (.5-1mg/kg). Research on exercise-specific benefits is limited, and higher doses increase risks without clear added benefit.

We discussed how personalized dosing can maximize the benefits of methylene blue. Understanding different administration methods and calculating an ideal dose tailored to your needs sets the stage for safe and effective supplementation. Emphasizing the mantra of starting low and going slow ensures a gradual introduction to methylene blue, allowing you to explore its potential confidently and cautiously.

Science Note on Dosage

- Methylene blue follows what scientists call a U-shaped dose–response curve:
    - At low to moderate doses, it supports mitochondria, boosts energy, and protects cells.
    - At high doses, the benefits flatten out or even reverse, sometimes creating more oxidative stress instead of less.

The safest and most effective results tend to come from the middle of the curve, not too little to be ineffective, and not so much that it backfires. The ranges in the table above are designed to keep you in that "sweet spot," consistent with both research and biohacking practice. Everyone is different and metabolizes differently, so we will once again emphasize the importance of listening to your body and intuition.

- Alzheimer's Disease

Unlike the weight-based ranges above, clinical trials in Alzheimer's disease have used fixed daily doses of methylene blue (or specialized formulations such as hydromethylthionine). Early studies suggested benefit around 138 mg/day. More recent re-analyses of Alzheimer's trials have shown that very low daily doses (8–16 mg/day) may be just as effective, and sometimes even more effective, because the body can only absorb a certain amount at once. In Alzheimer's research, it isn't about body weight or raw milligrams; it's about how much actually reaches the brain.

Safety Considerations and Who Should Avoid Methylene Blue

Methylene blue is generally safe when used at low doses, but there are specific situations where caution or avoidance is necessary. Please keep the following in mind:

- Serotonin Interactions: Do not combine methylene blue with medications that affect serotonin (such as SSRIs, SNRIs, or MAOIs) or with serotonin-boosting supplements (including 5-HTP, St. John's Wort, SAMe, or Rhodiola). Combining these can increase the risk of serotonin syndrome, a potentially dangerous condition. Methylene blue should also not be combined with psychedelics that act on serotonin receptors (such as psilocybin, LSD, MDMA, or DMT).
- G6PD Deficiency: Those with glucose-6-phosphate dehydrogenase deficiency should avoid methylene blue, as it can trigger hemolysis (breakdown of red blood cells).
- Pregnancy & Breastfeeding: Methylene blue is contraindicated in pregnancy due to the unknown risk to the fetus, and its safety during breastfeeding has not been established.

- Kidney Concerns: Those with impaired kidney function should use caution, as methylene blue may reduce renal blood flow and be eliminated more slowly.
- Other Medical Conditions: Anyone with chronic illness, complex medication regimens, or uncertain health status should consult a qualified healthcare provider before using methylene blue.

As with any supplement, it's wise to listen closely to your body. Signs such as dizziness, headaches, or agitation may indicate that your dose is too high or that your body needs a pause.

Tailoring Usage for Cognitive Enhancement

Achieving peak mental clarity requires more than finding the correct dose. Timing also matters. Take methylene blue 30 to 60 minutes before mentally demanding activities. This window gives the compound time to absorb and enhance cognitive function. Whether preparing for a high-stakes presentation, diving into a deep study, or working through a complex creative project, aligning your dosage with key moments of focus can amplify your mental performance. The synergy between methylene blue and your brain's natural rhythms may result in sharper concentration, heightened alertness, and a sense of presence that keeps you anchored in the task at hand.

When crafting your dosage protocol for cognitive enhancement, let your individual goals and current mental baseline be your guide. A typical starting point is ~0.23 mg per pound (0.5 mg per kilogram) of body weight, which is gradually increased based on your response. If you aim for more significant cognitive shifts, you can slowly build your dosage, but always with awareness. Your body will tell you what is working. Some people metabolize methylene blue quickly, while others may be more sensitive to its effects. Mindful experimentation helps you find your sweet spot without overstimulating your system.

To deepen the benefits, consider pairing methylene blue with brain-stimulating activities. Incorporate focused meditations, breath-work, puzzles, writing books, or neuroplasticity-based games into your routine. These intentional practices create a fertile environment that supports optimal brain performance. Over time, this consistency fosters short-term boosts and long-term cognitive resilience. Of course, safety always comes first.

Methylene blue provides a natural, science-backed approach to improved mental clarity. When used intentionally, at the right time, in the correct dose, and with proper care, it can become a powerful part of your cognitive wellness toolkit. The key is personalized adaptation: listening to your body, staying flexible with your plan, and making adjustments with patience and self-trust.

Remember, methylene blue is not a magic fix; it is one piece of a much larger puzzle. A truly optimized mind depends on sleep, movement, nourishment, nervous system regulation, and meaningful connection. When combined, these elements support a vibrant, sustainable form of cognitive health.

As you move forward, stay curious. Your journey with methylene blue is uniquely yours. Let it be a practice of tuning in, refining, and growing. With time, you may think more clearly, feel more focused, and inhabit a deeper presence in your daily life. The mind is not static. It is a living landscape; with the right tools, you can shape it into something extraordinary.

Dosage Considerations for Anti-Aging Benefits

With its unique ability to enhance mitochondrial efficiency, methylene blue holds promising anti-aging benefits. When considering doses specifically for anti-aging purposes, it is essential to recognize that these differ from those used for cognitive or athletic enhancement. Anti-aging protocols typically focus on sustaining cellular health over the long term rather than providing immediate performance boosts. A longevity-focused dosing approach involves sustained, moderate intake instead of sporadic high dosages. This consistent intake ensures that the body absorbs the compound effectively, promoting enduring mitochondrial support and minimizing oxidative stress over time.

Scientific investigations lay the groundwork for these recommendations. Studies suggest that a daily dose of ~0.113-0.23 mg/lb (0.25-0.5 mg/kg) of body weight (refer to dosage chart) effectively promotes cellular health and longevity. This dosage supports mitochondrial function without overwhelming the system, making it suitable for long-term use. It is important to remember that individual needs vary, so adjustments should be made based on personal health status and goals.

Pairing methylene blue with other anti-aging supplements can amplify its benefits. Consider combining it with antioxidants like CoQ10 or vitamin C to complement its role in combating oxidative stress. These combinations can produce a synergistic effect, enhancing overall cellular health. Resveratrol, another popular supplement, works well in conjunction with methylene blue, supporting similar pathways in cellular longevity. Such combinations provide a holistic anti-aging approach by targeting multiple mechanisms that contribute to cellular degeneration. You can create a powerful anti-aging stack tailored to your needs by thoughtfully selecting complementary supplements, which we will explore in more depth in the chapters to come.

Safety in long-term use is crucial when incorporating any supplement into your daily routine. With methylene blue, regularly monitoring your body's response is key to ensuring continued safety and efficacy. Note any changes in energy levels, skin tone, or other bodily functions potentially signaling a reaction. In the event of adverse effects, consider changing the dosage or cycling supplements to allow for a period of adjustment. Periodic healthcare provider check-ins can help keep you informed on your body's changing needs, ensuring methylene blue remains beneficial in your anti-aging strategy.

Sourcing high-quality methylene blue from reputable suppliers is crucial to ensure purity and safety. Opt for products that meet pharmaceutical-grade standards and avoid unnecessary additives to ensure optimal quality and purity. Proper storage is also vital; keep methylene blue cool and out of direct sunlight to maintain potency. By adhering to these guidelines, you can confidently incorporate methylene blue into your anti-aging regimen, allowing you to enjoy the potential longevity benefits while mitigating long-term risks associated with supplementation.

For those committed to aging gracefully and maintaining their vitality into later years, methylene blue offers a scientifically supported option for enhancing cellular health. Its role in optimizing mitochondrial function and reducing oxidative stress makes it invaluable in the quest for longevity. You can unlock its potential as part of a comprehensive anti-aging regimen by understanding dosage nuances and combining methylene blue thoughtfully with other supplements.

This approach supports physical health and contributes to mental well-being and overall quality of life as you age.

Patience and consistency are key to achieving health through the use of methylene blue. This compound's subtle yet profound effects manifest over time, gradually improving cellular health and vitality. Approach the process with openness and readiness to adapt based on bodily feedback. Through mindful use of methylene blue and complementary supplements, you can pave the way for a vibrant, healthy future with abundant energy and resilience.

By adopting a balanced methylene blue supplementation approach, you empower yourself to take control of the aging process. This perspective shifts the focus from merely adding years to adding life, to enhancing each moment with clarity, vitality, and strength. As research continues to uncover more about this remarkable compound's capabilities, its place in the constellation of anti-aging strategies solidifies, offering hope and opportunity for those living life to their fullest potential.

Optimizing Athletic Performance with Methylene Blue

Integrating methylene blue into your athletic regimen can be a transformative experience. It offers enhanced endurance, quicker recovery, and a deeper connection to your body's energy systems. When used intentionally, it becomes a powerful ally in both performance and recovery.

Timing is everything. For optimal results, take methylene blue approximately one hour before your workout. This gives your body time to absorb the compound and optimize cellular energy production as you step into physical exertion. Many athletes also find that a small post-exercise dose supports recovery, helping to reduce oxidative stress, ease muscle fatigue, and sustain energy levels throughout the day.

As mentioned earlier, methylene blue enhances mitochondrial efficiency at the cellular level, helping your cells produce energy (ATP) more effectively. With mitochondria operating at peak capacity, athletes experience increased stamina, improved oxygen utilization, and reduced lactic acid buildup, a key contributor to

soreness and fatigue. These effects are especially impactful during endurance sports or high-intensity training, where every ounce of energy matters.

Real-world routines show how athletes incorporate methylene blue into their protocols. A marathon runner, for instance, might take methylene blue with a complex carbohydrate-rich meal on the day before the race to support sustained energy. A professional cyclist can integrate it into their recovery routine, combining it with hydration, mineral replenishment, and stretching to minimize downtime between sessions. These examples demonstrate the versatility of methylene blue in achieving diverse athletic objectives.

Pay attention to your body's signals, especially in the early stages of use. Side effects, such as changes in blood pressure, fatigue, or headaches, may indicate that the dosage or timing needs adjustment. Hydration is essential when using methylene blue, as increased cellular activity can raise your body's need for water. Drinking enough fluids supports detoxification, muscle recovery, and overall metabolic health.

When used wisely, methylene blue can become a trusted part of your performance toolkit, helping you unlock new levels of energy, endurance, and resilience. Its benefits extend beyond the field or gym, supporting recovery, cellular vitality, and day-to-day wellness.

Ultimately, the value of methylene blue lies not just in its ability to boost performance but also in its support of a holistic approach to long-term health. Athletes who view their bodies as sacred instruments worthy of care, nourishment, and refinement find that methylene blue can amplify their connection to movement, purpose, and presence.

As more athletes discover its potential, methylene blue is emerging as a dynamic tool in the future of sports performance. Thoughtful integration now may become a standard of excellence for those committed to mastering their craft, both physically and energetically.

Safe Cycling: When and How to Take Breaks

Cycling supplements is a well-known concept among health enthusiasts. Strategically taking breaks allows your body to reset and maintain sensitivity to a supplement's effects. Methylene blue, like any compound, benefits from cycling. The idea is that intermittent use cessation prevents tolerance from developing, keeping benefits fresh and potent, and ensuring continued effectiveness. Cycling also reduces potential side effects, giving your system time to clear accumulated compounds.

Crafting a cycling schedule requires understanding your health goals and methylene blue's place in these objectives. For cognitive enhancement, a common approach involves five days on with two days off weekly, balancing steady support with regular breaks. Athletes may follow a distinct pattern, such as intensive use of methylene blue during training cycles and pausing during off- seasons. Longevity seekers may consider a monthly cycle: three weeks on, with one week off, to periodically cleanse and recalibrate mitochondrial functions.

Tailoring the cycle to your specific outlook optimizes benefits and minimizes body strain.

Recognizing when to take breaks is as crucial as cycling itself. Your body signals when it is time to pause. It may be time for a break if you're experiencing diminishing returns, where the benefits of methylene blue fade despite consistent use. Other indicators include unexpected fatigue, headaches, or changes in mood or sleep patterns. These suggest that your body needs rest.

Acknowledging these cues prevents overexertion of your system and maintains the long-term efficacy of methylene blue.

Effective cycling strategies encompass more than timing. During off periods, nurture recovery and balance through supportive practices. Engage in yoga or meditation to reduce stress and enhance well-being. Nutrient-dense foods rich in antioxidants support detoxification and cellular repair during methylene blue off- phases. Equally important, staying hydrated helps flush out residual compounds and improves cellular health. Implementing these lifestyle adjustments during cycling breaks boosts recovery, priming the body for when supplementation resumes.

Cycling methylene blue offers an opportunity to reassess your overall health strategy. Use this time to evaluate the fit of methylene blue within broader wellness goals. Reflect on its impact, noting areas for possible adjustments. This reflection guides approach refinements, ensuring the reintroduction of methylene blue aligns with evolving health objectives. Integrating these insights maintains a dynamic supplementation approach attuned to changing needs over time.

Cycling with awareness maximizes the benefits of methylene blue while safeguarding against overuse. This balanced approach supports long-term health, enhances the effectiveness of compounds, and ensures methylene blue remains a valuable part of your wellness toolkit. Understanding and applying cycling principles thoughtfully creates an environment in which methylene blue can work optimally without overwhelming the system.

Remember, cycling is about creating harmony within the body's systems, rather than just taking breaks. The rhythm of using and resting allows sustained benefits without overwhelming natural processes. As you explore the potential of methylene blue, consider how cycling can enhance your experience, offering both immediate advantages and long-term health benefits.

As you've seen, methylene blue's effects are powerful but depend significantly on how it's used. Personalized dosing, conscious timing, and cycling strategies form the foundation for a safe and effective experience.

In the next chapter, we'll bring it all together by exploring how to integrate methylene blue into your daily routine, anchoring it within your morning rituals, recovery practices, and energetic rhythms for long-term benefits.

Chapter 4

Integrating Methylene Blue into Daily Routines

Morning Rituals: Starting with Energy and Intention

Imagine the first light of dawn gently illuminating your room, signaling the birth of a new day. This quiet moment presents the perfect opportunity to incorporate methylene blue into your morning ritual. Starting your day with this compound can create a strong, energetic foundation, optimizing both mind and body for the day ahead. By supporting mitochondrial function, methylene blue enhances cellular energy and cognitive focus, laying the groundwork for clarity, presence, and vitality.

Creating a morning routine with methylene blue is both simple and deeply supportive. Upon waking, begin with hydration. Drink a full glass of water with lemon, along with some minerals, to reawaken your system and support optimal absorption. Then, take methylene blue using the delivery method that suits you best: a few drops in water, a sublingual lozenge, or a capsule. Follow this with a nutrient-rich breakfast filled with antioxidant-rich foods like berries, leafy greens, chia, or walnuts, and some protein, which complement methylene blue's ability to neutralize oxidative stress.

Pairing this with a grounding practice, such as meditation, breathwork, or gentle stretching, can further amplify your mental clarity and physical readiness. These practices help regulate the nervous system and prime the body for enhanced cellular energy benefits.

Timing is important. Cortisol levels naturally peak in the morning, helping you wake up and feel alert. Taking methylene blue during this natural energetic window allows it to synergize with your body's rhythm, enhancing its cognitive and energetic effects. A well-timed morning dose can transform groggy wake-ups into energized, focused beginnings, setting the tone for a productive and inspired day.

To further enhance the benefits of methylene blue, consider pairing it with other foundational supplements, such as vitamin D and omega-3 fatty acids, both of which support brain health and reduce inflammation. Creatine and L-Carnitine are two other supplements that pair well and help boost and sustain mental and physical energy.

Of course, consistency is key. Yes, busy mornings can present obstacles, so stay on track by preparing your supplements the night before and placing them beside your breakfast essentials. You can also set a gentle phone reminder to help you stay on track with your routine. These small cues help transform a habit into a ritual, making it easier to stay consistent even on hectic days.

Morning Visualization:

As you sip your water and take your morning dose, close your eyes. Imagine a blue light softly spreading through your body, igniting your cells, nourishing your energy, and aligning you with clarity. Let this inner light become a compass for the day ahead.

Morning Routine Checklist

- Hydrate: Start with a full glass of water. (with lemon & minerals)
- Supplement: Take methylene blue in your chosen form.
- Breakfast: Choose antioxidant-rich, nutrient-dense foods and protein.
- Mindfulness: Add meditation, breathwork, or stretching.
- Synergy: Pair with vitamin D, C, L-Theanine, Caffeine, and/or omega-3s for cognitive support.

By integrating methylene blue into your morning with presence and purpose, you cultivate a terrain where health and high performance thrive. You meet the day from a place of grounded energy, clarity, and calm readiness with one conscious choice at a time.

Enhancing Work/Life Performance: Focused, Present, and Energized

In today's fast-paced world, sustaining mental clarity and cognitive agility can feel like a constant balancing act. Methylene blue offers a promising solution for individuals seeking to maintain focus, energy, and mental resilience throughout the day. By enhancing mitochondrial efficiency in brain cells, methylene blue helps fuel sustained concentration and sharp decision-making. Imagine navigating a high-stakes meeting or creative project with a sense of presence and precision. That is the potential this compound offers when integrated with intention.

Timing and strategy are crucial for maximizing the benefits of methylene blue throughout your day. Consider taking your dose during a natural break, such as mid-morning or before a mentally demanding task. This window offers an opportunity to recharge and align the supplement's effects with your brain's cognitive rhythm. Pairing your dose with a brief mindfulness practice, such as deep breathing, a short walk, or even five minutes of stillness, can amplify its impact by calming the nervous system and enhancing clarity.

Real-world stories highlight the potential.

Sarah, a marketing executive juggling multiple projects, noticed a significant improvement in mental clarity and decision-making after incorporating methylene blue into her daily routine. Michael, an engineer working with complex data, reported reduced mental fatigue and increased focus during periods of high demand. Denia, an elementary school teacher on summer break, found herself with the stamina to complete a physically demanding gardening project in the southern heat, something she hadn't been able to do before. Mike, a retired veteran, shared that he felt both happier and lighter in his mood, describing a noticeable emotional lift. These experiences illustrate how methylene blue can transform mental output from scattered to streamlined, from foggy to laser-focused, and from physically unable to able, while also brightening the emotional outlook.

To support long-term success, create a personalized strategy. Visualize your day infused with quiet energy and unwavering focus. You start your morning with clarity, carry it through your day easily, and finish your tasks with a feeling of fulfillment. Methylene blue is not about overworking; it is about optimizing how you work, think, and show up. It offers a practical and inspiring tool for anyone seeking to enhance performance while promoting long-term well-being.

Fitness & Recovery: Fueling Movement and Cellular Repair

Imagine stepping onto the track or into the gym with a deep sense of readiness and inner power. Methylene blue can offer that competitive edge, enhancing performance well before muscle fatigue sets in. Supporting mitochondrial function enhances cellular energy production, allowing your body to train more effectively and recover more quickly. With more efficient energy output, muscles receive the oxygen and nutrients they need, reducing fatigue and enhancing overall performance. When used as a pre-workout supplement, methylene blue acts as a gentle yet potent energizer, priming the body for exertion and helping you confidently push your limits.

Timing is key. Taking methylene blue 30 to 60 minutes before your training session gives your body time to absorb it and begin amplifying energy pathways. Whether you're lifting weights, running hills, or cycling long distances, methylene blue can elevate your performance from the inside out.

But its influence does not stop there. Recovery is where methylene blue truly shines. After strenuous activity, your muscles experience micro-tears, inflammation, and oxidative stress. Methylene blue enhances blood flow and oxygen utilization, helping shuttle nutrients where they are needed most. This promotes muscle repair, reduces soreness, and speeds up recovery, allowing for more consistent training with fewer interruptions. Many athletes bounce back faster, train more frequently, and experience less stiffness and post-workout fatigue.

Hydration plays a vital role in maximizing the effects of methylene blue. Increased mitochondrial activity raises your body's fluid demands, so ensure you drink enough water, especially before and after training. Staying hydrated supports absorption and helps flush out the byproducts of intense exercise.

Whether you're chasing a personal best, building strength, or simply striving to feel more energized in your movement, this compound offers a scientifically grounded way to amplify your athletic journey. The key is intention. Tune into your body. Let your approach evolve. With thoughtful integration, methylene blue becomes more than a supplement; it becomes a supportive presence in your pursuit of physical vitality, endurance, and strength.

Evening Protocols: Rest, Recovery, and Circadian Alignment

As the day begins to slow and soften, preparing the mind and body for restful sleep becomes a sacred act of care. Methylene blue can serve as a gentle but powerful ally during this transition. By evening, cortisol levels naturally decrease, signaling your system to shift toward rest and repair. Introducing methylene blue at this time can support the body's movement into relaxation, calming the mind, reducing oxidative stress accumulated throughout the day, and helping you unwind more easily and gracefully.

Incorporating methylene blue into your nighttime ritual can be a grounding and restorative experience. Begin by creating a calming environment: dim the lights, turn off bright screens, and engage in a relaxing activity such as light stretching, meditation, or reading something soothing. About an hour before bedtime, take your methylene blue dose, ideally in a form that's easy to administer, such as a sublingual lozenge or liquid dropper. This timing allows it to work harmoniously with your body's circadian rhythm.

Pairing your dose with a warm, calming beverage can amplify the effects. Herbal teas, such as chamomile, lemon balm, or lavender, are perfect companions, enhancing the ability of methylene blue to relax both body and mind. The combination helps to ease the transition into a deeper, more restorative sleep.

Also, consider pairing methylene blue with other gentle evening supplements. Magnesium, known for its muscle-relaxing and calming effects on the nervous system, works synergistically to reduce tension and promote rest. Glycine, an amino acid with calming effects, may also be a helpful ally. It supports deeper sleep, lowers core body temperature, and assists in detoxification and neurotransmitter balance, making it a beautiful complement to methylene blue's oxidative stress-reducing qualities.

Of course, a busy mind and racing thoughts can challenge even the best intentions. Unprocessed emotions or overstimulation from the day can make it difficult to wind down. Establishing a consistent pre-sleep routine helps signal the body that it's time to rest. Simple practices, such as deep breathing, progressive muscle relaxation, or guided meditation, can work wonders. Journaling is another powerful tool, allowing you to release thoughts, clear mental clutter, and invite stillness.

Practical shifts in your environment can also support the evening effects of methylene blue. Keep your bedroom cool, dark, and quiet to encourage melatonin production and support your body's natural sleep-wake cycle.

Consider using blackout curtains, white noise, red light therapy, or an essential oil diffuser with calming scents, such as lavender or sandalwood, to help you relax. Limit screen time in the hour before bed; the blue light from devices can interfere with sleep hormones, undoing the relaxation you've worked to cultivate.

Evening Reflection Ritual

Use this simple checklist as a foundation to personalize your evening routine:

Set the Scene: Dim the lights (red light therapy is ideal) and play calming music.
Supplement: Take methylene blue with a soothing herbal tea.
Relaxation: Engage in meditation, breathwork, or gentle stretching. **Journaling:** Reflect and release your thoughts onto the page. List gratitudes from your day.
Optimize Environment: Adjust lighting (red-light therapy is ideal), temperature (cool it down), and minimize disruptions.

This evening ritual isn't just about improving sleep; it's about creating a container for wholeness. When you close your day with intention, your body feels safe to repair, your mind is free to soften, and your spirit can rest.

Sleep is not a passive act; it's a crucial regenerative process, especially for your mitochondria. During sleep, your body enters a state of repair: clearing out cellular waste, replenishing energy stores, regulating blood sugar, and calming inflammation. It's also when your brain consolidates memories and resets mood-regulating neurotransmitters. From a metabolic standpoint, poor sleep has been linked to insulin resistance, increased oxidative stress, and impaired mitochondrial function. In contrast, quality sleep enhances mitochondrial biogenesis and supports optimal cellular function. Combining methylene blue with intentional sleep practices can lead to improved rest and a greater investment in your long-term energy, mental clarity, and overall vitality.

Embracing methylene blue in your evening routine is a step toward holistic restoration. It supports your body in releasing the weight of the day while preparing you to rise renewed and resilient, which supports the anti-aging process. Let bedtime become a sanctuary, a sacred space where you can reset, receive, and reconnect with your natural rhythm of rest and replenishment.

Lifestyle Habits: Movement, Hydration, and Consistency

To truly unlock methylene blue's potential, your life environment, your movement, sleep, hydration, and habits must support it. The supplement itself is powerful, but it works best within a rhythm of intentional living.

Movement is a cornerstone of mitochondrial health. Regular physical activity, whether walking, yoga, dancing, running, cycling, or lifting, stimulates mitochondrial biogenesis and enhances circulation, oxygen delivery, and nutrient absorption. It complements methylene blue's mechanisms, amplifying energy production and performance.

Again, hydration is equally essential. Water facilitates nearly every cellular process, including the absorption of methylene blue and the transport of nutrients throughout the body. Aim for at least eight glasses of water daily (making sure to include minerals), adjusting the amount based on your activity level, climate, and individual needs. A well-hydrated body is a more efficient, more vibrant one.

Sleep, as discussed earlier, is a sacred pillar of mitochondrial repair. During rest, the brain and body detox, cells regenerate, and hormone systems recalibrate.

Without consistent, high-quality sleep, even the most targeted supplementation efforts may fall short. Methylene blue's benefits become magnified when paired with restorative sleep cycles.

When making changes, keep them simple and sustainable. Set gentle reminders to drink water. Track sleep with an App, and schedule time for joyful movement. Approach your lifestyle like a garden that requires presence, consistency, and gentle tending.

As you begin weaving methylene blue into your rhythms, waking with clarity, moving with power, unwinding with presence, you also step into a new level of discernment. Integration is not just about how you use a substance, but what you're truly inviting into your body. In a world where wellness shelves are saturated with options, learning to recognize quality becomes an act of self- honoring. This next chapter invites you into that sacred discernment. Because when it comes to methylene blue, purity matters. Potency matters. And most of all, trusting the source allows you to delve into the safety, alignment, and transformation this molecule was always meant to deliver.

Chapter 5

Evaluating and Selecting Quality Products

Finding a Brand You Can Trust

Methylene blue offers more than a quick fix. It speaks to the body's innate capacity for restoration and vitality. But with its growing popularity comes a flood of options. The shelves are crowded with bottles and tinctures, each claiming purity, potency, and precision. And while some products live up to that promise, others fall short of it. They may be diluted, contaminated, or lacking transparency. In this dynamic and sometimes overwhelming space, choosing a reputable brand is not just a matter of preference; it's a matter of safety, effectiveness, and alignment with your deeper healing journey.

Reputable companies take this sacred responsibility seriously. They invest in third-party testing to verify purity and potency. They provide transparent details about their sourcing and manufacturing processes. They support their claims with science and education, not just marketing. Most importantly, they honor the integrity of the compound itself, treating methylene blue not as a trend but as a powerful tool for transformation when used with care and respect.

Choosing a trusted brand supports your results and peace of mind. When you know what you're taking is clean, consistent, and consciously crafted, you can focus on tuning into your body's feedback and fine-tuning your journey. Many of these companies also offer thoughtful customer support, making the path feel less lonely and more empowered.

Recommended Brands to Explore

As we have discussed, purity and sourcing matter deeply when it comes to methylene blue. Not all products are created equal, and quality truly makes the difference between a trusted supplement and something that could do more harm than good. The following are companies I trust and recommend exploring. They have also earned respect in the biohacking and holistic health communities for their dedication to quality and integrity.

Troscriptions®

Troscriptions offers precision-dosed, pharmaceutical-grade methylene blue lozenges designed for optimal absorption and cognitive clarity. What sets them apart is their unwavering commitment to bioavailability, consistency, and science-backed formulation. Their products are developed with the guidance of medical experts and leading thinkers in the biohacking space, reflecting a deep respect for both efficacy and neurological integrity. Rather than overwhelming the body, Troscriptions focuses on intentional, clean delivery that supports peak performance, presence, and resilience.

Best365Labs

Best365 is a trusted and accessible brand offering high-purity methylene blue. They are praised for their transparency, affordability, and commitment to quality assurance, making them an excellent starting point for those embarking on their methylene blue journey. What sets Best365 apart is their thoughtful formulation of synergistic stacks, combining methylene blue with complementary ingredients for targeted support, whether for focus, mood, mitochondrial resilience, or detox. Their blends reflect a deeper awareness of how nootropics and wellness compounds can work together, offering users not just a product but a purpose-driven solution.

Optimal Health Systems (OHS)

Optimal Health Systems (OHS) has long been recognized for their integrity, transparency, and clinically formulated, whole-food-based supplements. I've personally used and trusted many of their products over the years and have consistently found them to be of the highest quality. Their newly launched methylene blue product, *Nano Blue*, reflects the same commitment to innovation, featuring advanced delivery technology that enhances absorption and cellular uptake. OHS brings care and research to everything they create. With Optimal Health System's philosophy of addressing root causes and supporting the body with nutrient-dense, bioavailable solutions, Nano Blue has the potential to bring methylene blue into a new era of accessibility and effectiveness.

Always remember that your body is unique, so while these are trusted companies, it's essential to trust your own experience and consult with a qualified practitioner when needed.

How to Choose with Confidence

Let your intuition and discernment work hand-in-hand with practical tools. Use this checklist when evaluating a brand:

- Third-Party Testing: Is the product independently tested for purity and potency
- Transparency: Does the company disclose sourcing, ingredients, and manufacturing processes?
- Do they publish or provide their COA without hesitation?
- Consumer Reviews: Do real users share consistent, trustworthy experiences?
- Customer Support: Is there guidance, care, and responsiveness if you have questions?
- Scientific & Energetic Integrity: Are claims backed by evidence, and is the company aligned with intentional, ethical practices?

The supplement market is noisy, but your path doesn't have to be. When you choose brands that honor both the science and the sacredness of this compound, you create an experience that is not just effective but energetically aligned. In the chapters to come, we'll continue exploring how methylene blue connects with more profound aspects of cognition, clarity, and transformation. But for now, remember: what you choose to put in your body matters. Making intentful choices is a form of devotion to your wellness, energy, and future self.

Purity, Potency, and Peace of Mind

In the world of supplementation, purity is a non-negotiable foundation. Ensuring purity isn't optional when working with compounds like methylene blue, especially those that influence mitochondrial function, brain chemistry, and redox balance.

It's essential.

Purity means the product is free from harmful contaminants that could compromise its safety and benefits. Impurities, such as heavy metals or leftover solvents, can cause adverse reactions or counteract the effects you seek. A pure methylene blue supplement performs as expected, delivering cognitive support, energy enhancement, and mitochondrial activation without hidden risks. It's important to understand that purity also reflects concentration. A product may be free of contaminants, but it won't produce the desired results if it lacks the expected potency. You want a supplement that provides consistent, clearly defined doses of methylene blue; no more, no less.

This leads us to potency, which refers to the strength or concentration of the active ingredient. A low-potency product may require higher doses to reach effective levels, increasing the potential for side effects. On the other hand, a well-dosed product supports efficacy at lower amounts, making it safer, more efficient, and often more cost-effective.

To assess both purity and potency, start with the label. Reputable brands clearly state the amount of methylene blue per serving, typically in milligrams (mg). Look for those that also include third-party testing certifications and symbols of transparency and trust, which confirm that the label's contents are accurately represented in the bottle. But labels can be misleading. Words like "pure" may be used loosely, without third-party validation or regulatory oversight. Always read beyond the front label. Search for a Certificate of Analysis (COA), a document showing the product has been tested for contaminants, potency, and identity.

Consider it a red flag if a company doesn't make this readily available. Be especially wary of products with vague descriptions, exaggerated claims, or unclear sourcing information. Overreaching marketing language often hides underwhelming formulations. When it comes to a compound as powerful as methylene blue, clarity and credibility matter.

Avoiding Hidden Toxins: What to Watch For

While methylene blue has remarkable potential for enhancing cognition, mood, and energy, not all products are created equal. Some carry unseen risks in the form of contamination, particularly heavy metals or leftover chemical solvents from poor manufacturing practices.

Common contaminants in methylene blue include lead, mercury, arsenic, and residual solvents like methanol or toluene. These impurities can have serious consequences: mercury and lead are known neurotoxins, and even trace amounts can accumulate in tissues over time, compromising neurological and metabolic function. Solvent residues may trigger nausea, dizziness, fatigue, or systemic toxicity. These risks run counter to the healing goals that methylene blue is meant to serve. That's why third-party testing is not optional; it's essential. Products tested by independent labs are screened for purity, potency, and safety. Look for labels that mention "USP Grade" or "Pharmaceutical Grade," both of which indicate high purity standards. Brands that offer COAs publicly on their websites demonstrate transparency and a commitment to consumer safety.

Safe purchasing practices include buying directly from the brand's website or authorized retailers, and avoiding third-party resellers whenever possible. Even more trustworthy are brands that formulate under USP (United States Pharmacopoeia) or cGMP (Current Good Manufacturing Practice) standards, which are recognized by health authorities for their quality control and consistency. Avoid falling for vague marketing or beautiful packaging that hides weak formulation. In this space, the details matter, and your health is worth that level of discernment.

Product Formats: Choosing the Right Delivery Method for You

Methylene blue is as versatile in form as it is in function. With a growing number of delivery formats available, users can choose a method that aligns with their lifestyle, preferences, and health goals. Whether you're new to methylene blue or a seasoned biohacker, understanding how these different forms work in the body can help you optimize both experience and efficacy.

Oral tablets are a familiar and convenient option, ideal for those who value structure and simplicity. These provide pre-measured doses that are easily incorporated into a daily supplement routine. Sublingual tablets, which dissolve under the tongue, offer faster absorption by bypassing the digestive tract, making them an excellent choice for those seeking a quick cognitive boost before mentally demanding tasks. Liquid drops are one of the most popular formats, prized for their dose flexibility and versatility. They allow fine-tuning based on your body's feedback and can be easily integrated into beverages or wellness routines. Though less common, powder forms appeal to those who love crafting customized supplement stacks and are perfect for smoothies or post-workout blends.

Each method carries unique qualities that influence absorption rate, ease of use, and bioavailability. For instance, sublingual delivery offers a faster onset by entering directly into the bloodstream, making it ideal for short-term mental clarity or energy boosts. In contrast, oral tablets move through the digestive system, which may slow the onset but provide a steadier release over time, beneficial for sustained energy and mitochondrial support throughout the day.

Liquid formats offer adaptability, especially for those experimenting with micro- dosing or titrating dosage levels. However, they often require more care and attention. Methylene blue can stain, so proper handling and storage matter.

Powders, although flexible, require proper mixing to ensure even distribution and effectiveness.

When choosing your ideal delivery method, consider a few key factors

- **Convenience:** How easily does it fit into your daily rhythm?
- **Speed of absorption**: Do you want rapid effects or a slow, sustained release?
- **Precision:** Do you want flexibility in adjusting your dose?
- **Ritual:** Do you enjoy blending your supplements into smoothies or wellness elixirs?

These questions guide what works and what feels good to you.

Examples: Finding What Fits

Everybody's life, goals, and preferences are different. Here are a few examples of how people tailor their delivery method to their daily rhythm:

Sarah is a busy professional who relies on sublingual tablets to sharpen her focus before important meetings. She appreciates the fast absorption and simple, no-water-needed convenience.

David prefers the steady support of oral tablets. He takes them with breakfast, integrating them seamlessly into his structured morning supplement regimen for sustained energy throughout the day.

Lisa, a wellness coach, loves liquid drops for their adaptability. She adjusts her dose based on her energy needs and adds it to herbal tea or smoothie bowls.

A fitness enthusiast, Michael mixes powdered methylene blue with his post- workout shake to support recovery and mental clarity after training.

These stories demonstrate how delivery formats aren't just functional but also personalized tools to support your rhythm, energy, and intention. As you explore the options, stay curious and responsive to how your body feels. What matters most is choosing a form that works harmoniously with your day-to-day life. Making it something you look forward to using, not something you forget or resist. Whether you're drawn to the immediacy of sublingual tablets or the simplicity of an oral capsule, the correct delivery method makes methylene blue effective and sustainable. Let your routine become a ritual. When you choose with awareness, your supplements become more than tools; they become allies.

Evaluating Supplier Credibility: Who You Buy From Matters

Choosing a methylene blue product is more than selecting a supplement; it's initiating a relationship with the company behind it. And, like any relationship, trust matters. A supplier's credibility directly impacts your safety, the effectiveness of your protocol, and your overall sense of empowerment throughout your wellness journey. Reputable suppliers operate with transparency and integrity.

They don't just sell a product. They support your health journey.

To help you make empowered, informed choices, here are key questions or red flags to explore before committing to a methylene blue brand:

- Do they provide third-party testing? Independent lab verification ensures the product is free of contaminants and contains the stated amount of active ingredient.
- Is a Certificate of Analysis (COA) available? A COA should be batch- specific and confirm purity, potency, and absence of harmful substances like heavy metals or residual solvents.
- Do they follow GMP or cGMP manufacturing practices? These are gold- standard protocols that ensure quality control and consistency across every bottle.
- Where do they source their raw materials? Transparency around sourcing shows care, ethics, and traceability.
- Do they provide detailed labeling and ingredient clarity? Vague language, such as "pure" without evidence, is a red flag.
- Can you access honest user feedback or professional reviews? Testimonials, case studies, and practitioner insights provide a grounded view of the product's performance in real-world applications.
- Is customer service responsive and informed? A trustworthy brand will engage with your questions openly and helpfully.
- Do they have exaggerated promises without research or references?

A Final Note on Supplier Integrity

Choosing a methylene blue product is a sacred act of self-support. Selecting a brand that honors the compound, its sourcing, and the consumer amplifies the potential benefits while minimizing risk. This is more than about purity and potency; it's about trusting the relationship you're entering with the company, the product, and your body.

Discernment is your ally. Ask the questions. Trust your intuition. Your mitochondria and your future self will thank you.

A Note from Nova

Thank you for journeying with me this far.

If you've made it to this point in Awaken with Methylene Blue, I imagine something is resonating, whether it's the science, the spirit, or the subtle nudges of your own intuition awakening.

This book was written as a bridge between the mystical and the measurable, the ancient and the emerging, the practical and the profound. And if any of that has sparked something within you, **I would be deeply grateful if you'd share your experience.**

Why Your Review Matters

When you take a moment to leave a review, you're doing more than just rating a book; **you're helping others discover a tool that could support their healing, expansion, and evolution.** Your words may be the exact frequency someone else needs to say yes to their next step.

Whether you're a health hacker, a healer, a curious soul, or simply someone exploring new ways to feel more alive in your body... your voice matters.

A Few Prompts to Guide Your Review:

- What inspired you to read Awaken with Methylene Blue?
- What surprised you the most, scientifically or spiritually?
- Did any rituals or protocols feel especially aligned?
- Who do you imagine would deeply benefit from this work?
- How has your relationship with your body, your brain, or your energy evolved since learning about methylene blue?
- Who would this book benefit most?

You can be brief. You can be poetic. You can be both. Just let it be real. Let it be yours.

Leave Your Review On:

With deep gratitude for walking this path alongside me, And thank you for sharing your light with others.

Nova L. Phoenix
author • guide • mitochondria whisperer • alchemist

Chapter 6

Smart Stacking, Synergy & What Sets Methylene Blue Apart

Introduction: Beyond a Single Molecule

While methylene blue shines brightly on its own, its potential amplifies when thoughtfully combined with complementary substances. This practice, known as stacking, is not about adding more for the sake of it. It's about resonance. Pairing methylene blue with the right companions can create a profound connection, especially when aligned with your individual goals.

This chapter explores those possibilities, weaving together practical science, spiritual alignment, and personalized optimization. We'll also look at how methylene blue stands apart from other nootropics and what you need to consider for safe, intelligent use - especially when combining supplements.

Smart Stacking: Aligning with Your Goals

Stacking is a tool. Like all tools, its impact depends on how and why you use them. Rather than mindlessly combining supplements, consider what you're truly seeking. Here are several intentional stack examples organized by desired outcomes:

Each of these stacks is more than a recipe; it's a conversation between molecules and intention. Choose what aligns with your current needs, and listen to your body as you experiment.

Mental Clarity & Focus

This trio blends stimulation with balance. Caffeine sparks alertness, while L-theanine softens the jittery edges, creating a smooth lift. Methylene blue enhances mitochondrial energy production, resulting in not only sharper but also longer-lasting and steadier clarity.

Mood & Calm Alertness

CBD and L-theanine both calm the nervous system while supporting a grounded emotional tone. Methylene blue layers in baseline cellular energy, gently lifting mood without overstimulation. This is a beautiful combination for those seeking presence, relaxation, and calm productivity.

Energy, Athletic Performance & Endurance

For the physically active, creatine replenishes muscular ATP, while cordyceps supports oxygen utilization and stamina. Methylene blue synergizes by enhancing electron transport in mitochondria, resulting in both increased output and faster recovery post-exertion.

Neuroprotection & Longevity

CoQ10 and methylene blue are both mitochondrial protectors, while omega-3 fatty acids ease neuroinflammation and support membrane health. Together, they create a stack that not only defends the brain but also encourages long-term resilience.

Deep Healing & Regeneration

Tissue and neurological repair require energy and signaling. Peptides such as BPC-157 or Dihexa support cellular recovery, while methylene blue fuels the mitochondria behind these processes. The result is a combination that nourishes regeneration at the deepest levels.

Hormonal Harmony & Stress Recovery

Methylene blue's mental stamina complements the stabilizing effect of adaptogens like ashwagandha and rhodiola. Add magnesium glycinate to soothe the nervous system, and this stack becomes a sanctuary for adrenal recovery and hormonal balance.

Anti-Aging & Longevity

Longevity is built on mitochondrial efficiency and resilience. Vitamin C helps recycle antioxidants, NMN replenishes NAD+, and methylene blue helps maintain the proper functioning of the electron transport chain. This trio supports both energy and graceful aging.

Detox & Cellular Renewal

Detox is not just about "removal" but about energy and replenishment. Methylene blue enhances mitochondrial detox pathways, glutathione recycles antioxidants, and CT-Minerals restore trace minerals often depleted in modern living. This stack supports both drainage and cellular renewal simultaneously.

Immune Resilience

Immune defense thrives on energy and balance. Methylene blue strengthens mitochondrial response, Vitamin D supports immune signaling, and zinc aids in viral defense and tissue repair. This stack is especially powerful during seasonal shifts or times of lowered immunity.

Table 2: Smart Stacking

Goal	Stack Components	Why It Works
Mental Clarity & Focus	Methylene Blue + Caffeine + L-Theanine	MB supports mitochondria and brain energy; caffeine stimulates; L-theanine smooths the stimulation.
Mood & Calm Alertness	Methylene Blue + L-Theanine + CBD	MB boosts cellular energy; CBD balances emotional tone; L-theanine reduces stress.
Energy, Athletic Performance & Endurance	Methylene Blue + Creatine + Cordyceps	Creatine supports muscular energy; cordyceps improves oxygen uptake; MB
Neuroprotection & Longevity	Methylene Blue + CoQ10 + Omega-3s	MB boosts mitochondria; CoQ10 recycles energy; omega-3s reduce neuroinflammation.
Deep Healing & Regeneration	Methylene Blue + Peptides (e.g., BPC-157, Cerebrolysin, or Dihexa)	Peptides support tissue and brain repair; MB enhances cellular energy to aid those processes.
Hormonal Harmony & Stress Recovery	Methylene Blue + Adaptogens (Ashwagandha, Holy Basil, or Eleuthero/Siberian Ginseng) + Magnesium Glycinate	MB provides mental stamina; adaptogens support adrenal balance and stress recovery; magnesium calms and nourishes the nervous
Anti-Aging & Longevity	Methylene Blue + Vitamin C + NMN or NAD+ Precursors	Vitamin C supports antioxidant recycling; NMN boosts NAD+; MB enhances mitochondrial function & electron transport for resilience.
Detox & Cellular Renewal	Methylene Blue + Glutathione + CT-Minerals	MB drives mitochondrial detox; glutathione recycles antioxidants; minerals replenish what's lost during detoxification.
Immune Resilience	Methylene Blue + Vitamin D + Zinc	MB enhances cellular defense; Vitamin D supports immune signaling; zinc aids repair

Smart stacking is about synergy, not rigidity. The stacks you've just explored are invitations to experiment, not prescriptions to follow dogmatically. Every body is unique, and what resonates for one person may feel too stimulating or too subtle for another. As you explore, let curiosity and intuition guide your choices. Notice how your energy, focus, and mood shift. Remember, the real magic isn't just in the supplements themselves, but in how they interact with your lifestyle, your inner rhythm, and your commitment to listening to your body's wisdom.

Pro Tip: Stacks aren't the whole picture; think of them as blueprints. Pairing any of these with supportive practices, such as sauna, rebounding, yoga, breathwork, or simply staying well-hydrated, can amplify their effects. These lifestyle enhancers help your body move energy, detoxify, and integrate the benefits of each stack more deeply.

Safety Considerations: Stacking with Wisdom

Even the most beneficial compounds can cause an imbalance when used excessively or without awareness. Methylene blue is generally safe at low doses, but certain combinations require caution. For a comprehensive overview of who should avoid methylene blue and potential interactions, refer to the safety considerations in Chapter 3.

Watch for Serotonin Interactions

Because methylene blue has mild monoamine oxidase (MAO) inhibitory effects, which can impact serotonin metabolism, caution is advised when stacking it with SSRIs, SNRIs, or other serotonin-boosting medications.

Prescription Medications to Use With Caution:

- SSRIs (e.g., fluoxetine, sertraline, citalopram, escitalopram)
- SNRIs (e.g., venlafaxine, duloxetine)
- MAOIs (e.g., phenelzine, tranylcypromine)
- Serotonin-Boosting Supplements to Use With Caution:
- 5-HTP
- L-tryptophan
- St. John's Wort
- SAMe
- Rhodiola Rosea (mildly serotonergic)
- MDMA, psilocybin, and other serotonergic psychedelics

When in doubt, pause, research, and consult with experts. The risk of serotonin syndrome is rare at low doses but should never be overlooked. This is where discernment becomes protection. Safety is the foundation of sustainable transformation.

Keep Your Stack Clean

Use high-purity, third-party tested supplements. Avoid unnecessary fillers or mystery blends. The combinations you're seeking come from clarity, not clutter.

What Sets Methylene Blue Apart

Among today's vast array of cognitive enhancers, methylene blue stands apart for its unique and effective mechanism of action. Rather than overstimulating neurotransmitters like many nootropics, it works on a deeper, more foundational level as an electron cycler supporting mitochondrial respiration.

By facilitating efficient electron transfer within the mitochondria, methylene blue enhances ATP production while simultaneously reducing oxidative stress, a byproduct often linked to aging and neurodegeneration. This rare combination of energy amplification and cellular protection makes methylene blue a standout: it not only fuels the brain but also protects it from damage.

Dr. Chris Palmer, author of Brain Energy, emphasizes that mitochondria aren't just the "powerhouses of the cell"—they are essential to life itself. If mitochondrial energy production halts, life ceases within minutes. Methylene blue's support at this level positions it as a foundational wellness tool.

Expanding the Systemic Benefits of Methylene Blue

While methylene blue is often celebrated for its cognitive-boosting properties, its reach extends far beyond the brain. This molecule enhances cellular energy production and reduces systemic oxidative stress, offering benefits that impact stamina, resilience, skin health, and longevity.

Emerging studies suggest that when applied topically, it may promote collagen synthesis and protect against oxidative skin damage, making it a promising candidate for anti-aging skincare and regenerative protocols.

From Brain to Body: A Holistic Wellness Molecule

What began as a compound studied for its effects on memory and mental stamina is now being explored for its role in optimizing the entire body. Its anti- inflammatory effects, mitochondrial support, and antioxidant capacity make methylene blue a multidimensional wellness tool that supports recovery, energy regulation, and graceful aging from the inside out.

In Summary: What Truly Sets It Apart

Amid a crowded field of nootropics, methylene blue occupies a unique space:

Mechanism: Unlike most nootropics that act via neurotransmitter stimulation (like caffeine or racetams), Methylene Blue works at the cellular energy level, specifically in the mitochondria.

Dual Action: Methylene blue enhances ATP production and reduces oxidative stress. This is something few compounds can do simultaneously.

Systemic Impact: While many nootropics are brain-specific, methylene blue affects all high-energy tissues, including the heart, muscles, brain, and more.

Legacy and Science: Backed by 100+ years of research, with current clinical interest surging in cognitive aging, neurodegeneration, and mitochondrial dysfunction.

It is not a stimulant, yet it enhances clarity. It's not an antioxidant in the traditional sense, yet it neutralizes oxidative stress with precision. Its multidimensional benefits make it not just a supplement, but a paradigm shift.

A Gentle Reminder: Personalization is Key

Your journey is your own. Some people thrive on small, consistent microdoses. Others prefer to cycle or use methylene blue only in focused windows. Trust your intuition. Track your experience, reflect regularly, and be willing to adapt as your needs shift.

Final Reflection

As we've explored, stacking methylene blue with other supportive tools can be a game-changer. One that amplifies cognitive function, enhances resilience, and deepens your relationship with vitality itself. And it's not just personal experience: respected voices from the field, from researchers to integrative physicians to leading biohackers, are echoing these possibilities. Yet even with such promising feedback, misinformation and fear still cloud the conversation. In the next chapter, we'll gently dispel these myths and bring light to the lingering doubts and misconceptions that surround methylene blue. It's time to move from confusion to clarity so that you can walk this path with grounded confidence, scientific insight, and intuitive trust in your body's wisdom.

Chapter 7

Debunking Myths & Addressing Safety with Methylene Blue

A Bridge Between Skepticism and Empowered Use: Seeing Through the Fog

Even with so many respected voices now speaking openly about methylene blue (from neuroscientists to integrative oncologists to leading biohackers), myths, half-truths, and misunderstandings still swirl around this little blue molecule. Perhaps that's inevitable. Any time something ancient is rediscovered and reintroduced into modern practice, it's met with both awe and suspicion. Some dismiss methylene blue as a fad, a passing wellness craze that will fade as quickly as it appeared. Others whisper fears about safety, side effects, or "blue urine", letting headlines overshadow decades of research. And still others mistakenly assume it is either too powerful or too trivial, missing the reality of how it works within the body.

This chapter is about cutting through that noise. We'll examine the most common myths and misconceptions surrounding methylene blue, setting them alongside both the science and personal experiences. By doing so, you'll be able to separate hype from truth to make your own empowered, informed choices. Because the truth is simple: Methylene blue is neither a miracle cure nor a dangerous gimmick. It is a tool. And like any tool, its power lies in how and why it is used. Here, we provide you with the grounded insight you need to determine if, and how, this tool aligns with your path toward clarity, vitality, and overall well- being, both mentally and physically.

Myth 1: "It's Just a Textile Dye"

Yes, methylene blue was first synthesized as a dye in the 19th century. And yes, its bright color still turns heads. But to reduce it to "just a dye" is to ignore more than a century of profound medical use.

Methylene blue's bold blue hue made it invaluable in biology labs, helping scientists visualize cells under microscopes. But its real leap into medicine came when the FDA approved it as a treatment for methemoglobinemia, a rare condition in which the blood's ability to carry oxygen is impaired.

Over time, its clinical applications expanded. Methylene blue has been used to:

- Reverse cyanide and carbon monoxide poisoning
- Support recovery from vasoplegic shock in surgeries
- Treat chronic urinary tract infections
- Alleviate symptoms of bipolar disorder and other mood conditions (via mitochondrial and neurotransmitter pathways)

Its vibrant past is not a disqualifier; it's a doorway into a long, validated history of therapeutic potential.

Myth 2: "There's No Scientific Evidence"

This is the most pervasive myth and the easiest to dispel.

Methylene blue has been studied for decades in respected fields such as:

- Neuroprotection
- Mitochondrial energy metabolism
- Cognitive performance
- Anti-aging and oxidative stress regulation

Its role as an electron cycler enables it to facilitate more efficient cellular respiration. This is not speculative; it's a biochemical fact. Studies have confirmed methylene blue's ability to cross the blood-brain barrier, reduce oxidative stress, and enhance ATP (adenosine triphosphate, or energy) production at the cellular level.

Its cognitive and neuroprotective effects have also been explored in models of Alzheimer's, Parkinson's, and traumatic brain injury.

Bottom line: Methylene blue is not a trendy supplement with a shaky foundation; it is a compound deeply rooted in decades of peer-reviewed science.

Myth 3: "It's Unsafe"

Used responsibly, methylene blue has a strong safety record, especially at low doses.

Hospitals continue to use it regularly, both intravenously and orally. When used as a supplement or nootropic in microdoses (typically .23mg -.45 mg/lb or 0.5–1 mg/kg of body weight), side effects are rare and generally mild.

Most common temporary reactions include:

- Blue-green urine or stool discoloration (harmless but surprising)
- Mild gastrointestinal discomfort when taken on an empty stomach
- Slight headaches or brain fog when taken in too high a dose

More serious risks arise when:

- It's combined with SSRIs or serotonergic medications (risk of serotonin syndrome)
- The product is low-quality or contaminated
- Doses are taken far beyond what's recommended

This chapter, and this book, are dedicated to safe and intentional use, because clarity is your greatest protection.

Myth 4: "It Affects Mood Negatively"

Actually, many users report mood elevation and emotional clarity while using methylene blue. There are emerging clinical studies that suggest low-dose methylene blue may also aid in treating residual depressive and anxiety symptoms in bipolar disorder when used alongside standard mood stabilizers, without evidence of triggering mania.

This is likely due to its mitochondrial support and mild MAO-inhibiting properties, which can enhance serotonin and dopamine tone. While more research is still needed, early studies suggest it may be helpful in mood disorders and neurodegenerative diseases.

That said, methylene blue should never be combined with SSRIs, SNRIs, or other serotonergic compounds without medical oversight.

Myth 5: "It's Only for Professionals or Biohackers"

Some people feel intimidated, thinking they need a PhD in biochemistry or a stack of bloodwork to use methylene blue. Not so.

With proper education, discernment, and attention to dosage and quality, anyone can safely explore the benefits of this substance. This book is your guide—not just for understanding the science, but for developing a respectful, empowered relationship with the compound.

Knowledge and intuition are your best tools. Start low, listen often, and let your body lead the way.

Safety Rooted in Science, Reinforced by Experience: Clinical and Scientific Endorsements

Experts like Dr. Michael Hamblin, a leader in photomedicine, and Dr. Francisco Gonzalez-Lima, a neuroscientist and pioneer in methylene blue research, have highlighted its neuroprotective, mitochondrial-enhancing, and photodynamic properties.

Far from being unorthodox, their research has appeared in The Journal of Neuroscience, Frontiers in Cellular Neuroscience, and Scientific Reports— solidifying the role of methylene blue in evidence-based medicine.

Real-World Wisdom: Stories from the Field

- Emma, a creative entrepreneur, experienced mild headaches when starting. By lowering her dose and staying hydrated, the discomfort passed, and she felt sharper than ever.
- Dominick, a college student healing from a concussion, used methylene blue as part of a neurorehabilitation protocol. His energy, word recall, and mood steadily improved.
- Lisa, a single mom and caregiver, used low-dose methylene blue to reduce burnout and mental fatigue. Within weeks, she felt more resilient and emotionally balanced.

These are not isolated anecdotes. They represent a pattern: when used intentionally, methylene blue becomes a supportive ally for body, brain, and spirit.

Navigating Information Overload

In today's wellness landscape, information is everywhere: marketing claims, fragmented science, flashy packaging. It can feel overwhelming to know what (or who) to trust. Learning to discern is one of the most important skills you can develop on this journey.

Trustworthy sources include:

- **PubMed** for peer-reviewed studies
- **Harvard Health Publishing** for accessible medical overviews
- **ResearchGate.net** for direct access to scientific papers
- **Researchers like Francisco Gonzalez-Lima and Michael Hamblin** for pioneering work in mitochondria and photomedicine
- **Functional medicine podcasts or summits** where clinicians share real-world insights
- **Practitioner case studies and integrative protocols** grounded in lived patient outcomes

At the same time, be wary of exaggerated claims, supplements without transparency around purity testing, or companies that prioritize branding over evidence. The goal isn't to become skeptical of everything, but to develop the discernment to separate noise from wisdom so that you can move forward with clarity and confidence.

Voices From the Field: Perspectives on Methylene Blue

Now that we've dispelled the myths and misconceptions, it's worth pausing to hear how others are contributing to this evolving conversation. Across neuroscience, integrative medicine, and the biohacking community, methylene blue is being recognized not as a fleeting trend but as a serious and versatile tool for cellular health. These voices add perspective and depth, reminding us that what you've just read is part of a much larger movement toward reclaiming energy, clarity, and resilience.

Gary Brecka ~ Human Biologist & Biohacker

"Methylene blue isn't a trend. It's a tool. And those who understand how mitochondria drive human performance are paying attention."

Brecka emphasizes pharmaceutical-grade purity and highlights methylene blue as a mitochondrial ally—enhancing ATP production, improving oxygen utilization, and supporting resilience.

Dr. Francisco Gonzalez-Lima ~ Neuroscientist, University of Texas at Austin

With decades of research, Gonzalez-Lima has demonstrated that low-dose methylene blue functions as an electron cycler in the mitochondria, maintaining energy flow even under stress. His work demonstrates methylene blue's ability to improve memory, enhance learning, and protect the brain against oxidative damage. He describes methylene blue as enhancing "brain cytochrome oxidase activity, improving memory functions, and providing neuroprotection."

Dr. Tony Jiménez ~ Integrative Oncologist, Founder of Hope4Cancer

At Hope4Cancer clinics, methylene blue is incorporated into IV therapy protocols as part of a terrain-based approach to healing. For Dr. Jiménez, supporting the environment in which cells thrive is just as crucial as addressing disease itself. His clinical use of methylene blue reflects its growing acceptance in integrative oncology, from neurological support to aiding recovery.

Dr. Scott Sherr, MD ~ Functional Medicine & Mitochondrial Health

Dr. Sherr highlights methylene blue's broad potential for those struggling with low cellular energy:

"About 95 percent of people have some level of mitochondrial dysfunction, and methylene blue has the potential to help most of them … It could be used across the board for a variety of patients to help them feel better and faster."

His words position methylene blue not just as a performance enhancer, but as a practical support tool for everyday energy and resilience.

Tim Gray ~ UK's Leading Biohacker & Founder of the Health Optimisation Summit

Gray has experimented with methylene blue as part of his cognitive and longevity routines. His advocacy in the UK wellness space has helped bring Methylene blue into broader awareness, positioning it as a supplement that sharpens focus, supports mitochondrial health, and complements other biohacking practices.

Brian Probst ~ Founder of Blue Brain Nootropics

As the founder of Blue Brain Nootropics, Probst has brought pharmaceutical-grade methylene blue into the nootropics mainstream, championing it as one of the most effective cognitive enhancers available. He emphasizes its ability to sharpen focus, stabilize mood, and protect the brain under oxidative load. His advocacy has introduced methylene blue to a broad audience of biohackers seeking both mental performance and neuroprotection.

Why These Voices Matter

Together, these perspectives create a powerful chorus: methylene blue is being explored by researchers, clinicians, and biohackers alike. Whether in the lab, the clinic, or the optimization community, the message is the same: methylene blue is not a fad. It is a versatile, evidence-based tool with the potential to transform our understanding of energy, cognition, and cellular health.

Replacing Fear with Wisdom

You don't need to be an expert to use methylene blue. You just need to be curious, informed, and willing to listen to your body.

Let go of fear-based stories. Replace them with discernment, practice, and reverence for your body's innate intelligence.

The myths are just noise. You now have the tools to see clearly, choose wisely, and move forward from a place of grounded empowerment.

Reflection Prompt

- What story, if any, about methylene blue were you carrying before reading this chapter?
- What feels different now?
- What other stories, about your health, your capacity, your potential, are ready to be rewritten as well?

Looking Ahead

We've cleared away the myths, misunderstandings, and fears that have surrounded methylene blue throughout history. Along the way, we've heard from trusted voices in the field who are affirming its value. Together, these perspectives remind us that methylene blue is not just a molecule of the past but a living key to the future, one we are only beginning to understand.

Chapter 8
Future Directions in Methylene Blue Research

With the myths dispelled and the doubts cleared, we can finally look forward with fresh eyes. What emerges is a key that may help unlock the future of medicine, longevity, and human potential. Across research labs and integrative clinics, methylene blue is emerging as more than a supportive tool of the present; it is a glimpse into what's possible when we align cellular wisdom with scientific innovation. This chapter invites you to imagine a future where energy, clarity, and resilience are not fleeting states but the foundation of a new era of vitality.

A Glimpse Into the Future

Imagine walking through the corridors of a futuristic wellness center, where personalized protocols harness light, frequency, and molecular precision to regenerate vitality from the inside out. In this vision, methylene blue isn't just a compound; it's a central player in a paradigm shift toward cellular optimization, mitochondrial rejuvenation, and integrative healing.

Science is catching up with what some have intuitively felt: that healing begins in the cell, and methylene blue may be one of the keys.

Mitochondria at the Forefront

At the heart of methylene blue's power lies its elegant influence on mitochondria, the microscopic engines within every cell that generate ATP, our body's primary source of energy. Emerging research confirms what biohackers, athletes, and forward-thinking physicians have observed: when mitochondrial function is optimized, so is everything else.

Methylene blue acts as an electron cycler, supporting the flow of electrons through the respiratory chain. This improves ATP production while simultaneously reducing reactive oxygen species (ROS). These unstable byproducts contribute to aging and cellular damage. The result? Greater energy efficiency, reduced oxidative stress, and a stronger cellular foundation for healing, performance, and longevity.

However, perhaps even more compelling is the fact that methylene blue may stimulate mitochondrial biogenesis, the process by which new mitochondria are created. This means it's not just helping existing cells function better; it may help regenerate your internal energy infrastructure.

Neuroprotection and Regenerative Potential

Few areas of research have generated as much excitement as the potential role of methylene blue in preventing and supporting neurodegenerative diseases.

Early-stage studies suggest that it may help reduce the formation of tau tangles and beta-amyloid plaques, both hallmarks of Alzheimer's disease. It also appears to protect against neuron loss, improve cognitive performance, and enhance cellular metabolism in the brain.

In models of Parkinson's disease, stroke, and traumatic brain injury, methylene blue has shown potential in reducing neuroinflammation and promoting neurological repair. While more human trials are needed, the signals are strong: Methylene blue may one day become a core element of integrative cognitive care.

A New Frontier in Healing Rare Disorders

Mitochondrial disorders like MELAS syndrome or Leigh syndrome, once considered medically intractable, are now being studied through the lens of redox modulation and mitochondrial repair. Researchers are investigating how methylene blue may provide metabolic stabilization and energy restoration in these challenging cases, bringing hope where little existed before.

Whole-Body Optimization: Inflammation, Longevity & Graceful Aging

Methylene blue's influence extends far beyond the brain. Systemically, it has shown the ability to modulate inflammation, influence the Nrf2 antioxidant pathway, and reduce chronic oxidative stress, a root cause of many degenerative diseases.

Conditions such as autoimmune disorders, arthritis, long COVID, and even fibromyalgia may benefit from this combination of mitochondrial support and anti- inflammatory effects. Additionally, methylene blue's ability to reduce advanced glycation end products (AGEs) may make it a valuable ally in promoting skin health, vascular protection, and metabolic wellness.

In the realm of longevity, its dual action, protecting existing mitochondria while encouraging new mitochondrial growth, makes it one of the most compelling tools for those seeking not just a longer life, but a more vital one.

Alzheimer's & Cognitive Decline

Among the most closely studied applications of methylene blue is its potential role in addressing neurodegenerative diseases, particularly Alzheimer's.

Research has shown methylene blue's ability to reduce the formation of tau tangles and beta-amyloid plaques, both of which disrupt neuronal communication and are hallmarks of Alzheimer's pathology. Derivatives such as LMTX have entered clinical trials, showing hints of cognitive improvement and slowing of disease progression.

Beyond protein aggregation, methylene blue also enhances mitochondrial function and cerebral blood flow, offering a multi-layered approach to brain health. Dr. Francisco Gonzalez-Lima's work has demonstrated that methylene blue improves memory and learning in both animal and human studies by boosting cytochrome oxidase activity in neurons. He describes it as *"a cognitive enhancer with neuroprotective properties,"* pointing to its potential future role in integrative cognitive protocols, offering hope in the early stages of Alzheimer's and other dementias.

Dosing in Alzheimer's Disease

The history of methylene blue in Alzheimer's disease has produced seemingly conflicting results, with both "high" and "low" doses showing up in the science. An early clinical trial suggested that around 138 mg/day could slow decline in people with moderate Alzheimer's. However, in 2019, researchers reanalyzing two major trials found that participants on what was intended to be a "control" dose of just 8 mg/day were actually experiencing measurable cognitive and brain-structure benefits. Their modeling suggested that ~16 mg/day may be the optimal dose when methylene blue is used alone.

A 2022 follow-up review confirmed this surprising finding: it's not the sheer size of the dose that matters, but how much of the compound actually makes it into the bloodstream. Because absorption saturates at higher doses, more milligrams don't always mean more benefit. This is why low-dose strategies (8–16 mg/day) are now taken seriously in Alzheimer's research, even though the field still considers methylene blue investigational.

Post-COVID & Chronic Fatigue Syndromes

The global pandemic has left millions with lingering symptoms. Fatigue, brain fog, and dysautonomia are often described as "long COVID." Increasingly, researchers point to mitochondrial dysfunction and redox imbalance as underlying drivers of this condition. Here, methylene blue may have a unique role.

By improving electron flow in the mitochondria, methylene blue can support energy production where it has faltered. Its antiviral properties, long recognized in blood transfusion safety, add another dimension, as does its ability to regulate nitric oxide, which is often dysregulated in post-viral fatigue. Emerging interest suggests methylene blue could be studied as part of integrative recovery protocols for long COVID, post-viral syndromes, and even myalgic encephalomyelitis/chronic fatigue syndrome (ME/CFS). While the research is still in its early stages, the potential is profound: a molecule that restores vitality in the aftermath of viral disruption.

Arthritis & Autoimmune Inflammation

Chronic inflammation is a root driver of many age-related and autoimmune conditions, and here, too, methylene blue shows promising results. Studies indicate that methylene blue can downregulate NF-κB, a master switch of inflammation, while simultaneously activating the Nrf2 pathway, which triggers the body's own antioxidant defenses. In animal models of arthritis, methylene blue has been shown to reduce joint swelling, protect cartilage, and improve mobility.

These dual actions, which calm excessive inflammation while energizing mitochondria, make methylene blue a promising candidate for conditions such as rheumatoid arthritis, lupus, and fibromyalgia. Early indications also suggest it may mitigate oxidative stress in vascular and connective tissue, pointing toward potential benefits in systemic autoimmune and inflammatory disorders. Though clinical validation is still needed, methylene blue may one day support a new kind of integrative rheumatology: one that treats not only symptoms but the mitochondrial and energetic roots of disease.

Bipolar Disorder

Emerging clinical studies have explored methylene blue as an adjunctive treatment in bipolar disorder, particularly for residual depressive and anxiety symptoms that sometimes remain despite mood stabilizers. Early findings suggest potential benefits without evidence of triggering mania, a crucial safety consideration. However, this research remains preliminary and limited to small, short-term studies. While intriguing, this area of application should be approached with medical supervision until larger, long-term trials provide more precise guidance.

Expanding Horizons: Photodynamic & Integrative Oncology

Beyond neuroprotection and longevity, methylene blue is also emerging in the field of integrative oncology. In photodynamic therapy, methylene blue can act as a light-activated agent, selectively targeting dysfunctional cells when paired with specific wavelengths of light.

Clinics like Hope4Cancer, led by integrative oncologist Dr. Tony Jiménez, are beginning to explore methylene blue as part of terrain-based healing protocols. This approach doesn't view methylene blue as a standalone cure, but rather as part of a broader system that creates a biological environment where healing can take root. The fusion of light, frequency, and molecular medicine points to a horizon where methylene blue could become a cornerstone of innovative cancer care.

The Research Landscape: Where We're Headed

Scientific interest is exploding, with multiple clinical trials now investigating methylene blue in areas such as:

- Alzheimer's disease and mild cognitive impairment
- Post-COVID fatigue and brain fog
- Athletic performance and metabolic health
- Autoimmune and inflammatory modulation
- Skin aging and topical regeneration
- Mood & Biopolar Disorder

Table 3: Potential Applications

Focus Area	Key Findings	Potential Applications
Mitochondrial Support	Increases ATP, Improves electron flow, reduces ROS	Chronic Fatigue, mitochondrial disorders, Energy optimization, recovery, fatigue, althetic performance.
Neurodegeneration	Reduces tau, boosts neuron survival, improves memory, reduces neuroinflammation	Alzheimer's, Parkinson's, brain aging prevention
Mitochondrial Biogenesis	Stimulates new mitochondria, supports repair	Healthy Aging, Longevity, resilience, cognitive repair, peak performance
Inflammation Modulation	Reduces inflammatory markers, protects against oxidative damage	Autoimmune disease, brain fog, arthritis, long COVID, mood & brain health
Age Related Decline: Skin and Tissue Health	Supports collagen, reduces cellular damage & aging, improves skin elasticity, preserves cognition	Anti-aging skincare, wound healing

As we move forward, methylene blue's ripple effects extend from the cellular level, supporting not just mental clarity and physical energy but also the body's innate capacity for healing.

While many of methylene blue's most promising applications are already being studied in areas like neuroprotection, inflammation, and longevity, research is also branching into new and sometimes unexpected directions. Some of these frontiers are still in their early stages. Still, they offer a glimpse into how this small molecule could play a role in future innovations across medicine, wellness, and technology.

Table 4: Emerging & Experimental Applications of Methylene Blue

Application Area	Potential Benefits	Research Status
Septic Shock	Modulates nitric oxide pathways and supports blood pressure regulation	Early-stage clinical use
Nanotechnology Delivery*	Improves targeting and bioavailability through nano-formulations	Early development stage
Antimicrobial Use	Explored in sanitizers and non-toxic preservation methods	In vitro testing + product development
Neural Plasticity	Possible support for synaptic growth and cognitive recovery	Early exploration; limited human trials

* What is Nanotechnology?

Nanotechnology operates at the tiniest scale imaginable; a nanometer is one billionth of a meter. In supplements and medicine, this often means creating *nano-formulations* where compounds are packaged into microscopic carriers. For methylene blue, this could help protect the molecule, improve its absorption, and even target it more precisely to tissues such as the brain or mitochondria. Think of it like giving methylene blue a tiny spaceship to travel in, shielding it until it arrives exactly where it's needed most.

These surprising applications remind us that methylene blue's story is still unfolding. From critical care to targeting delivery systems, it continues to reveal possibilities far beyond what we've already explored. As research expands, we are only beginning to glimpse the full spectrum of what this small blue molecule may offer to our overall healthspan.

Closing Words

Methylene blue is no longer hiding in the shadows of medical obscurity. It is stepping into the light; honored by history, validated by science, and welcomed by a community of empowered users. The future isn't just about biohacking. It's about remembering that true vitality begins within, and that our cells are ready to respond when given the right tools.

Final Reflection: A Threshold of Possibility

So here we are, at the threshold of something bigger than just supplementation.

Methylene blue invites us into a new way of thinking about energy, healing, and vitality, a way that is simultaneously cellular, spiritual, scientific, and intuitive. It reminds us that healing is not about chasing quick fixes, but about meeting the body where it is, and helping it remember its original blueprint.

Whether you're recovering, optimizing, or simply curious, you are standing in a doorway of what's possible.

What would it look like to live in a body that feels alive, clear, and supported from the inside out?

What doors could open if you treated your mitochondria, not as tiny engines, but as sacred sparks of life?

This is your invitation.

The next chapter... begins with you.

A Note from Nova

Thank you for journeying with me this far.

Now that you've completed *Awaken with Methylene Blue*, I hope that the words have become more than information; they've become an invitation into your own next chapter.

This book was written as a bridge between the mystical and the measurable, the ancient and the emerging, the practical and the profound. And if any of that has sparked something within you, **I would be deeply grateful if you'd share your experience.**

Why Your Review Matters

When you take a moment to leave a review, you're doing more than just rating a book~ you're **helping others discover a tool** that could support their healing, expansion, and evolution.

Your words may be the exact frequency someone else needs to say yes to their next step.

Whether you're a health hacker, a healer, a curious soul, or simply someone exploring new ways to feel more alive in your body... your voice matters.

A Few Prompts to Guide Your Review:

- What inspired you to read *Awaken with Methylene Blue*?
- What surprised you the most—scientifically or spiritually?
- Did any rituals or protocols feel especially aligned?
- Who do you imagine would deeply benefit from this work?
- How has your relationship with your body, your brain, or your energy evolved since learning about methylene blue?
- Who do you feel this book would benefit most?

You can be brief. You can be poetic. You can be both.

Just let it be real. Let it be yours.

Leave Your Review On:

With deep gratitude for walking this path alongside me,

And thank you for sharing your light with others.

Nova L. Phoenix
author • guide • mitochondria whisperer • alchemist

Reader's Resources

As you've discovered, methylene blue is more than a supplement; it's a doorway into new ways of thinking about energy, resilience, and vitality. If you'd like to explore further, here are some trusted resources for continuing your journey.

Trusted Brands

- Troscriptions® — https://www.troscriptions.com Precision-dosed lozenges designed for cognitive clarity and clean delivery. Reader Discount: https:// troscriptions.com Use code NOVALIGHT for 10% off.
- Best365Labs — https://www.best365labs.com Accessible, high-purity methylene blue and thoughtfully formulated stacks.Reader Discount: Use code NovaLight for 10% off.
- Optimal Health Systems (OHS) — https://www.optimal-healthsystems.com/#code=KVZLOVE Whole-food-based supplements and Nano Blue innovation, reflecting OHS's deep commitment to root-cause

wellness. (No discount code available, but purchases made through my professional account help support my work.)

Note: I did not select these companies due to partnerships. I discovered and trusted them first, and only later formed professional connections with some of them. They are included here because I value their integrity and the quality of their products.

Podcasts & Learning

- Smarter Not Harder Podcast (Troscriptions® / Dr. Scott Sherr) Nootropics, functional medicine, and mitochondrial health.
- Best365labs— News & Media
- Optimal Health Nutrition- Health & Research Blog
- Health Optimization Podcast with Tim Gray: Biohacking, resilience, and longevity.
- Gary Brecka Interviews: Performance and Practical Applications of Methylene Blue.
- Lectures by Dr. Francisco Gonzalez-Lima: Groundbreaking research on brain energy metabolism.

Research & Exploration

- PubMed.gov — Peer-reviewed studies on methylene blue across cognition, energy, and health.
- Integrative medicine forums & biohacking communities — Active discussions on safe and creative methylene blue applications.

References

- Alzheimer's Drug Discovery Foundation. (2021). Methylene blue – Cognitive Vitality for Researchers. Retrieved from https://www.alzdiscovery.org/cognitive-vitality
- APC Pure. (n.d.). What is USP grade? A methylene blue 1% case study https://apcpure.com/news/what-is-usp-grade-a-methylene-blue-1-case-study
- Blue Brain. (n.d.). Improving sports performance with methylene blue https://blubrain.co.uk/enhancing-sports-performance-methylene-blue
- Callaway, E. M., & Xue, H. (2018). From mitochondrial function to neuroprotection: The role of methylene blue. Journal of Neurochemistry, 144(6), 697–711 https://doi.org/10.1111/jnc.14288
- Compass Laboratory. (n.d.). Methylene blue https://compasslaboratory.com/en-ie/blogs/news/methylene-blue
- Delaney, K., & Brown, A. (2024). Methylene blue. In StatPearls. StatPearls Publishing https://www.ncbi.nlm.nih.gov/books/NBK557593/
- Dempsey, T. (n.d.). What is methylene blue? A look at its surprising health benefits https://drtaniadempsey.com/what-is-methylene-blue-a-look-at-its-surprising-health-benefits
- Eden Health. (n.d.). Methylene blue dosage: Guidelines for safe & effective use https://www.tryeden.com/post/methylene-blue-dosage
- Fagron Academy. (n.d.). Pharmacogenetics – Basics and implications in the future of personalized medicine https://www.fagronacademy.us/blog/pharmacogenetics---basics-and-implications-in-the-future-of-personalized-medicine
- Gillman, P. K. (2006). A review of serotonin toxicity data: Implications for the mechanisms of serotonin syndrome. Psychopharmacology, 187(3), 389–403 https://doi.org/10.1007/s00213-006-0416-z
- Gonzalez-Lima, F., & Auchter, A. M. (2015). Protection against neurodegeneration with low-dose methylene blue and near-infrared light. Frontiers in Cellular Neuroscience, 9, 179 https://doi.org/10.3389/fncel.2015.00179

References

- Gonzalez-Lima, F., & Bruchey, A. K. (2010). Neurometabolic mechanisms for memory enhancement and neuroprotection of methylene blue. Progress in Neurobiology, 92(3), 193–206 https://doi.org/10.1016/j.pneurobio.2010.06.004

- Gonzalez-Lima, F., & Meineke, D. E. (2016). Methylene blue as a neuroprotective agent. Progress in Neurobiology, 137, 69–85 https://doi.org/10.1016/j.pneurobio.2015.12.007

- Internal Healing & Wellness MD. (n.d.). Methylene blue protocol: Health & longevity breakthrough https://internalhealin gandwellnessmd.com/the-methylene-blue-protocol-a-breakthrough-for-health-and-longevity/

- Li, Q., et al. (2020). Effect of long-term methylene blue treatment on the cognitive and pathological changes in an Alzheimer's disease mouse model. Aging, 12(22), 22793–22809 https://doi.org/10.18632/aging.104100

- LongevLab. (n.d.). The new health color for biohackers: Methylene blue! https://www.longevilab.com/en/the-new-health-color-for-biohackers-methylene-blue

- Marques, M. B., & Mayfield, C. A. (2014). Methylene blue in the treatment of methemoglobinemia. Transfusion Medicine Reviews, 28(2), 74–81 https://doi.org/10.1016/j.tmrv.2013.12.003

- Nair, N. P. V., & Gudelsky, G. A. (2004). Serotonin syndrome: Role of the 5-HT2A receptor in the mechanism of toxicity. Behavioural Brain Research, 147(1–2), 49–54 https://doi.org/10.1016/j.bbr.2003.09.022

- Neuroveda Health. (2024, September 30). Rev up your mitochondria, the powerhouses of your cells https://www.neurovedahealth.com/post/let-s-talk-about-your-mitochondria

- Oz, M., Lorke, D. E., & Petroianu, G. A. (2009). Actions of methylene blue and its derivatives on cellular functions. Progress in Neurobiology, 87(3), 145–170 https://doi.org/10.1016/j.pneurobio.2009.01.007

- PCCA. (n.d.). Methylene blue: From textile dye to potential clinical wonder https://www.pccarx.com/Blog/methylene-blue-from-textile-dye-to-potential-clinical-wonder

- Pharmacist Consult. (2024, January 8). Methylene blue: Pharmacist review | 2024 update [Video]. YouTube https://www.youtube.com/watch?v=wGPMWTWL_xA

References

- Pillai, V. B., & Rajamohan, S. B. (2023, June 16). Targeting mitochondrial dysfunction using methylene blue. bioRxiv https://doi.org/10.1101/2023.06.16.545146

- Pillai, V. B., & Rajamohan, S. B. (2024). Targeting mitochondrial dysfunction using methylene blue: Mechanistic insights and therapeutic potential. Journal of Translational Medicine, 22(1), 45 https://doi.org/10.1186/s12967-024-05002-8

- Preston, T. L., & Gonzalez-Lima, F. (2014). Therapeutic benefits of methylene blue on cognitive function. Neurobiology of Learning and Memory, 114, 23–34 https://doi.org/10.1016/j.nlm.2014.05.001

- Rock Ridge Pharmacy. (n.d.). Methylene blue: Shining a light on its cognitive-enhancing effects https://www.rockridgepharmacy.com/methylene-blue-shining-a-light-on-its-cognitive-enhancing-effects

- Rojas, J. C., Bruchey, A. K., & Gonzalez-Lima, F. (2012). Methylene blue and neurodegeneration: A critical review of the evidence. Current Medicinal Chemistry, 19(8), 1122–1132 https://doi.org/10.2174/092986712799320557

- Schelter, B. O., Akuffo, O. K., Corrigan, F., et al. (2019). Effect of hydromethylthionine on cognitive decline and brain atrophy in Alzheimer's disease: A reanalysis of two randomized controlled trials. Journal of Alzheimer's Disease, 71(2), 535–547 https://doi.org/10.3233/JAD-190484

- Shin, H. J., Lee, S. M., & Park, S. H. (2022). Clinical effectiveness and prospects of methylene blue. Precision and Future Medicine, 6(1), 14–21 https://doi.org/10.23838/pfm.2022.00079

- Shirley, R. A., & Sinha, A. (2014). PharmGKB summary: Methylene blue pathway. Pharmacogenetics and Genomics, 24(3), 133–138 https://doi.org/10.1097/FPC.0000000000000024

- Tree of Light Health. (n.d.). Methylene blue: The magic bullet for cellular health, neuroprotection, and athletic performance https://treeoflighthealth.com/methylene-blue-the-magic-bullet-for-cellular-health-neuroprotection-and-athletic-performance/

- Troscriptions. (2022, October 6). Epigenetic modulation (diet, exercise, methylene blue, and more) https://troscriptions.com/blogs/main/epigenetic-modifications

- Wainwright, M., & Crossley, K. B. (2002). Methylene blue—a therapeutic dye for all seasons? Journal of Chemotherapy, 14(5), 431–443 https://doi.org/10.1179/joc.2002.14.5.431

References

- Wainwright, M., & Crossley, K. B. (2016). Methylene blue: The long and winding road from stain to therapeutic agent. Biochemical Pharmacology, 122, 56–65 https://doi.org/10.1016/j.bcp.2016.09.005
- Wainwright, M., & Crossley, K. B. (2022). Review on methylene blue: Its properties, uses, toxicity and applications. Water, 14(2), 242 https://doi.org/10.3390/w14020242
- Walter-Sack, I., Rengelshausen, J., Oberwittler, H., Burhenne, J., Mueller, O., Meissner, P., & Mikus, G. (2009). Methylene blue— Absorption, metabolism, and excretion in humans and comparison with other species. Journal of Pharmacy and Pharmacology, 61(5), 587–595 https://doi.org/10.1211/jpp/61.05.0005
- Wen, Y., Li, W., Poteet, E. C., Xie, L., Tan, C., Yan, L. J., Ju, X., Liu, R., Qian, H., Marvin, M. A., Goldberg, M. S., She, H., Mao, Z., Simpkins, J. W., & Yang, S. H. (2011). Methylene blue improves mitochondrial function and reduces oxidative stress in fibroblasts from progeria patients. Aging Cell, 10(6), 957–969 https://doi.org/10.1111/j.1474-9726.2011.00738.x
- Wischik, C. M., Staff, R. T., Wischik, D. J., Bentham, P., Murray, A. D., Storey, J. M. D., & Harrington, C. R. (2022). Tau aggregation inhibitor therapy: Development of hydromethylthionine in Alzheimer's disease. Journal of Alzheimer's Disease, 89(1), 291–312 https://doi.org/10. 3233/JAD-220077
- Xue, H., & Yang, S. H. (2021). The potentials of methylene blue as an anti-aging drug. Aging and Disease, 12(6), 1449–1463 https://doi.org/ 10.14336/AD.2021.0414
- Yadav, N., et al. (2019). Nootropic nanocomplex with enhanced blood–brain barrier permeability for the treatment of neurodegenerative disorders. International Journal of Pharmaceutics, 563, 324–335 https://doi.org/10.1016/j.ijpharm.2019.04.054
- Zheng, X., Zhang, Y., Zhang, X., Li, Y., Zhao, Y., & Ma, X. (2017). Anti-aging potentials of methylene blue for human skin longevity. Scientific Reports, 7, 2475 https://doi.org/10.1038/s41598-017-02419-3
- Zhu, Y., Carvey, P. M., & Ling, Z. (2017). Methylene blue extends lifespan and improves mitochondrial function in a mouse model of aging. Aging Cell, 16(2), 330–341 https://doi.org/10.1111/acel.12562

www.ingramcontent.com/pod-product-compliance
Lightning Source LLC
Chambersburg PA
CBHW071531120626
46550CB00006B/2415